"Healing and living your best life with cancer is not only possible but achievable thanks to the author's essential insights for newly diagnosed cancer patients. This wonderful guide book clearly gives cancer patients a fantastic roadmap towards wellness from a holistic perspective. I wish I had such an empowering resource when I was diagnosed myself. I hope this book will be found in the office of every Integrative practitioner, GP and Oncologist."

Justine Laidlaw - The Natural Bird
Colon Cancer Survivor, Integrative & Functional Medicine Cancer Coach

....

"I have always been intrigued by the practice of Kintsugi—where something broken is made whole and even more beautiful. Many facing cancer, myself included, have experienced this first hand. Paul blesses us by baring his cracks of grief and loss by filling them with the gold of personal experience and global collaboration to tell a story of hope and healing. This concise, scientifically informed, and thoughtfully presented guide is a gift to us all."

Dr Nasha Winters
Author: The Metabolic Approach to Cancer

....

"Winston Churchill said 'Men occasionally stumble over the truth, but most of them pick themselves up and hurry off as if nothing had happened'. Paul McKenna was actually propelled into the reality of cancer through his partner's illness. Rather than 'hurrying off', Paul has honed the many truths they learnt into this well-crafted book. As a cancer survivor myself, and one who has spent time with many others working on transforming the disease, I highly recommend Empowering Hope."

Dr Ian Gawler OAM
Books include: You Can Conquer Cancer and Blue Sky Mind.
App: Allevi8   iangawler.com

....

"In the cancer journey we can feel alone and broken. Having a roadmap to find ourselves and put ourselves back together (maybe better than before) is a great gift. This book is such a gift. Use it to find yourself, heal, live, love, and connect." Di x

Di Foster
Mentor, Speaker & Storyteller

....

When you are diagnosed with cancer, your whole world is shattered - physically, mentally, spiritually and emotionally. Finding your healing pathway can be daunting, confusing and overwhelming. Empowering Hope by Paul Mckenna is a wonderful foundation to connect the pieces back together again - rebuilding a new life filled with gratitude and love - the glue that holds everything together.

Cathy Brown
Author: My Answer to Cancer

....

"Being confronted with a serious, life-threatening diagnosis such as cancer is a huge shock that everyone experiences in a very different, traumatic way. There is one thing that most people have in common, though: Resorting to the internet in a desperate attempt to learn more, find ways of dealing with the diagnosis and, hopefully, a plan to not only survive but also thrive for as long as possible after treatment. Unfortunately, online investigations usually result in feelings of overwhelm, panic and even despair. Having a resource such as Paul McKenna's "Empowering Hope" is a much more effective, gentle and supportive way of obtaining an evidence-based, realistic and actionable roadmap that covers the basic healing principles. The survival stories and additional resources provide additional inspiration and hope, which is another important cornerstone of every cancer journey. Thank you for creating this beautifully illustrated book, Paul!"

Patricia Daly
Nutritional Therapist (dipNT, mBANT, rCNHC), Ocular Melanoma (stage 3c) survivor
Author: The Ketogenic Kitchen (co-written with Domini Kemp, a melanoma and breast cancer survivor)

....

2

You can believe the diagnosis,
not the prognosis

Deepak Chopra

Book design, illustrations, photography (unless specified) by Paul McKenna

Edits by Deb Hoadley

empowering.au

ISBN 978-0-6450804-3-8 (hardback)
ISBN 978-0-6450804-4-5 (paperback)
ISBN 978-0-6450804-5-2 (ebook)
ISBN 978-0-6450804-6-9 (audiobook)

CONTENTS

INTRODUCTION

An Evidence-based Natural Approach to Cancer

'Empowering Hope: Natural, Evidence-Based Cancer Approaches' is your trusted roadmap for managing cancer naturally, offering a holistic and evidence-backed approach that can also complement standard medical treatments. It believes in the incredible capacity of your body to heal itself, even when facing chronic or seemingly incurable diseases like cancer.

There's a growing focus in medical treatments on enhancing the immune system's ability to fight and eliminate cancer cells. This guide aligns with this progressive approach, embracing a holistic method that considers your mind, body, and spirit. Its goal is to reduce anxiety, stress, and inflammation while strengthening your immune system's capacity to combat cancer.

This empowering combination equips your body to not only manage but, in some cases, overcome cancer. Letting go of suppressed emotions is a powerful step towards finding peace and healing.

In the world of cancer, there are countless paths to healing, and choosing natural methods may offer the best long-term results.

This approach is not about leaving things to luck; it's about making healthy choices right from the moment of diagnosis, choices that may play a pivotal role in recovery, achieving remission, or simply leading a healthier life as you navigate the challenges of illness.

A natural approach will take time and effort, especially in the early stages, but it's a path well worth taking. Early intervention is vital, as cancer can become too complex to overcome if left unchecked. Remember, knowledge is power, and hope is a wellspring that can sustain you.

Perhaps most importantly, find joy in your life and discover enjoyable ways of living. This will sustain you and guide you toward full health. Trust in yourself and your intuition.

Naturally, I wish you all the best on your journey to healing and empowerment.

Success is the sum of small efforts - repeated day in and day out

Robert Collier

I'm not a medical doctor. Nor do I provide medical advice. The information provided here is evidence-based and looks at both established and emerging science and research. Please make careful decisions about your treatment and journey forward.

It always seems impossible until it's done

Nelson Mandela

SO YOU HAVE CANCER...

You Have Time to Think

Facing a cancer diagnosis can be overwhelming, prompting numerous questions and a sense of dread. It's essential not to rush into treatment decisions based on fear-driven urgency. Take the time to assess your situation, try to understand why you might have cancer, and carefully consider the best approach.

Chemotherapy and medications can negatively impact the microbiome and immune system.[1-2] Long-term cancer survivors who have had invasive or aggressive conventional treatments report reduced quality of life.[3-4] Immunotherapy and targeted therapies can have negative impacts on the immune system, including autoimmune reactions, immunosuppression, and endocrine effects that are not easily reversible. Recurrence of cancer is possible even after conventional treatments.

A Natural Approach

Prioritise immune support through a natural, sustainable approach. Strengthen your immune system, reduce inflammation, and minimise oxidative stress.[5] These side-effect-free approaches may offer enhanced long-term effectiveness, contributing to overall well-being, better relationships, and stress reduction.

Stay patient and conduct regular testing to ensure you're on the right track.

Where do I Start?

Begin by calming yourself and carefully considering all aspects of your situation.

Breathe!

Two safe and effective treatments supporting immune system health are crucial to your initial cancer journey. Intravenous Vitamin C (IVC) and Fecal Microbiota Transplant (FMT) are explained in more detail in the following pages. IVC enhances immune function and reduces cancer growth, particularly when the immune system is fully functional.[6] Chemotherapy or other treatments may damage and reduce the effectiveness of the immune system. FMT, involving the transfer of healthy fecal microbiota, aims to rebalance the gut flora, playing a pivotal role in immune health.[7]

Integrate ongoing healthy lifestyle changes tailored to your needs. Start with simple practices like walking and focusing on slowing your breathing. Consider incorporating yoga, as it can prove highly beneficial both in the short and long term. Focus on eating a large variety of healthy, whole foods, fruits and veggies to boost your immune health. Rely on your intuition to make decisions that lead to the best life outcomes, emphasising thoughtful choices for your long-term well-being.

HOLISTIC
Approaches

Holistic approaches contribute to an overall improved quality of life for cancer patients. They may also provide comfort and relief from treatment-related side effects. Emphasising the mind-body connection, holistic approaches like mindfulness, yoga, and meditation play a pivotal role in managing stress and anxiety during cancer treatment.

Patients actively engage in their care by adopting lifestyle changes that empower them to promote overall health, providing relief from physical and emotional symptoms such as nausea, pain, and muscle tension induced by conventional treatments. Aligned with personal beliefs, these practices reflect cultural, spiritual, or individual perspectives, highlighting a comprehensive approach to health and healing.[1-2]

Standard medical approaches often fall short in supporting holistic mind, body, and spirit approaches. Practices such as Traditional Chinese Medicine, Ayurveda, or other indigenous healing methods may be overlooked despite their potential effectiveness. Although these ancient practices may lack extensive scientific validation, individuals often find value in their holistic approach.

Long-term health considerations significantly influence a cancer patient's choice of treatment, as certain standard medical treatments may lead to significant side effects and long-term health issues, potentially resulting in a lower quality of life.

The adoption of emerging and potentially effective cancer treatments into standard medical practice can be a prolonged process due to factors such as complexity, ethical considerations surrounding extensive clinical trials, reluctance to change, and resistance to and downgrading of holistic approaches. This delay may result in patients being offered outdated practices that are less effective.

Faced with a cancer diagnosis and a short prognosis, patients may explore alternative options in the hope of achieving a better long-term positive outcome.

Holistic approaches, rigorously applied from the early stages, may prove more effective against cancer over the long term and with fewer side effects. They also promote lifelong health and well-being benefits.

CANCER MANAGEMENT *Roadmap*

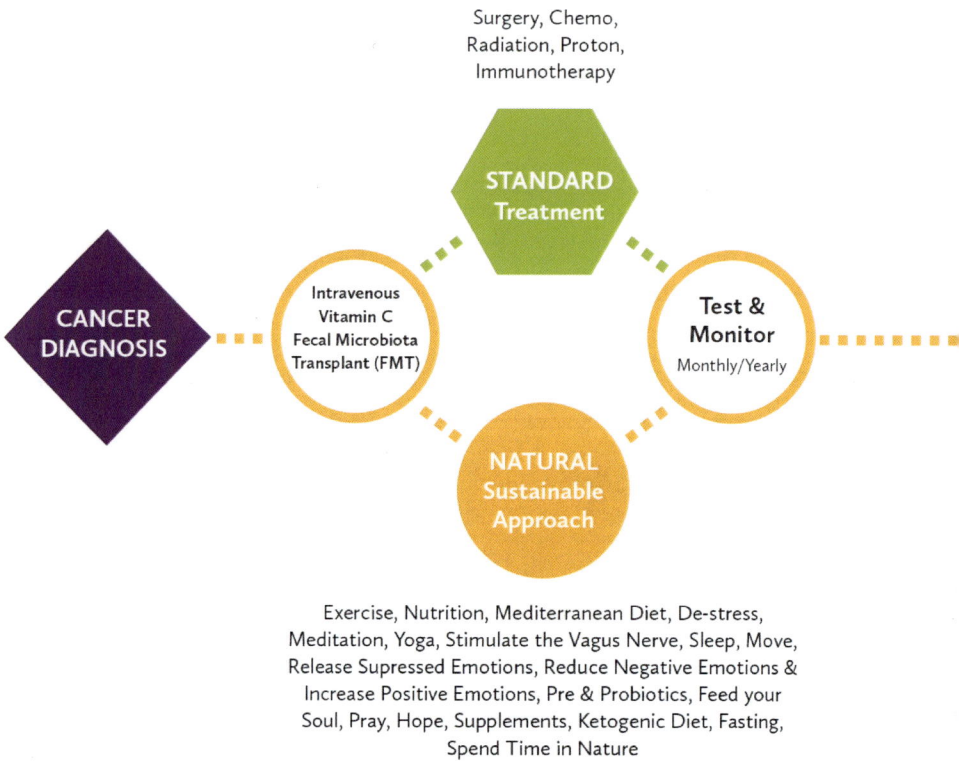

Surgery, Chemo,
Radiation, Proton,
Immunotherapy

STANDARD Treatment

CANCER DIAGNOSIS

Intravenous
Vitamin C
Fecal Microbiota
Transplant (FMT)

Test & Monitor
Monthly/Yearly

NATURAL Sustainable Approach

Exercise, Nutrition, Mediterranean Diet, De-stress,
Meditation, Yoga, Stimulate the Vagus Nerve, Sleep, Move,
Release Supressed Emotions, Reduce Negative Emotions &
Increase Positive Emotions, Pre & Probiotics, Feed your
Soul, Pray, Hope, Supplements, Ketogenic Diet, Fasting,
Spend Time in Nature

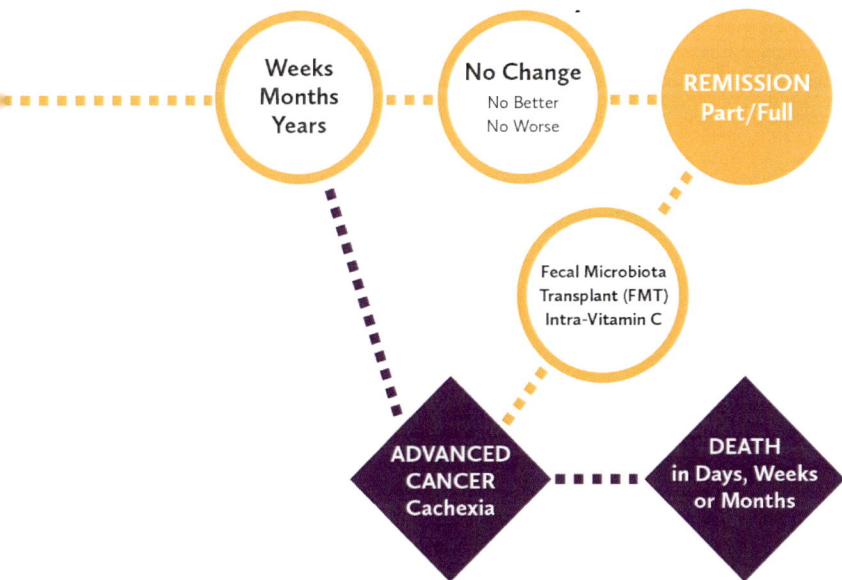

INTRAVENOUS VITAMIN C (IVC)

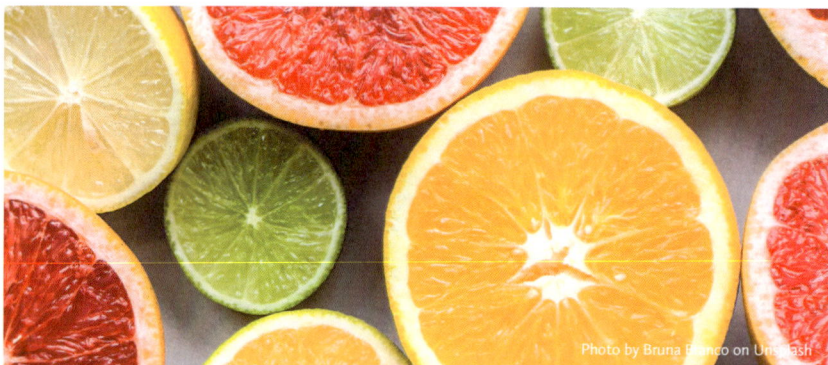

Photo by Bruna Branco on Unsplash

Playing a pivotal role in immune system support, vitamin C significantly contributes to the production and functionality of white blood cells, crucial defenders against infections and illnesses. This highlights the vitamin's importance in fortifying the body's natural defence mechanisms. Additionally, vitamin C is indispensable for collagen synthesis, a vital protein providing structure to connective tissues, skin, blood vessels, and bones. This dual role in immune function and tissue maintenance underscores the vitamin's significance in supporting overall bodily resilience.[1]

Intravenous vitamin C (IVC) is a method that enables rapid and efficient absorption into the body, having a considerable impact on cancer cells through targeted and elevated concentrations. Research and clinical studies have indicated that high doses may selectively induce cell death in cancer cells[2], sparing normal cells through mechanisms like hydrogen peroxide generation.

Importantly, IVC is most effective when the immune system is fully functional.[3] Treatments such as chemotherapy can damage the immune system function and therefore reduce the benefit of IVC.

Furthermore, intravenous administration enables higher and sustained blood levels of vitamin C compared to oral supplementation, particularly advantageous in cancer treatment where achieving therapeutic tissue concentrations is crucial. This potential increase in tissue concentrations may contribute to the anti-oxidative and immune-modulating effects of vitamin C, creating an environment supportive of the body's natural defence mechanisms against cancer.

Intravenous vitamin C is considered safe when administered and closely monitored by qualified healthcare professionals.

FECAL MICROBIOTA TRANSPLANT *(FMT)*

The gut microbiome, a diverse community of microorganisms residing in our digestive tract, plays a crucial role in shaping the effectiveness of our immune system. Operating as a protective barrier, it shields against the intrusion of harmful pathogens into the bloodstream. Essential to the development and maturation of immune cells, the microbiome ensures a strong and coordinated response to potential threats.

By producing anti-inflammatory substances, such as short-chain fatty acids, these microorganisms contribute to maintaining a balanced and appropriate immune response. Moreover, the gut microbiome engages in competitive exclusion, out-competing harmful pathogens for resources and thwarting their establishment. Nurturing a diverse and healthy gut microbiome through dietary habits is vital for sustaining optimal immune function and overall well-being.

In the realm of cancer, the gut microbiome undergoes significant alterations, impacting its composition and diversity, leading to disruptions and potential dysbiosis or systemic inflammation.

Addressing this, Fecal Microbiota Transplant (FMT) involves transferring fecal microbiota from a healthy donor into the intestine of a cancer patient, aiming to restore balance.

This ancient Chinese medical practice, dating back at least 1700 years, positively influences the immune response and contributes to the overall well-being of individuals undergoing cancer treatment.

Emerging research indicates FMT stands as a promising avenue for rebalancing the gut microbiome and enhancing the immune system particularly in response to cancer.[1-2]

Start With IVC and FMT

Both IVC and FMT treatments offer significant benefits in boosting immune system function and have the potential to reduce cancer growth and development, making them an ideal starting point.

IVC is most effective when your immune system is fully functioning, ideally before chemotherapy. Both IVC and FMT are considered safe when administered by qualified professionals and are highly supportive of any subsequent treatments, whether they be standard medical treatments or holistic approaches. These treatments may prove highly effective in managing your cancer.

CANCER MANAGEMENT *Plan*

A passive approach to cancer alone may prove ineffective. The body requires a combination of both gentle and intense physical activity to achieve peak fitness and health.[1] The most benefits are derived from combining exertion with mindfulness.[2-3] Consider it akin to certain yoga poses—physically demanding yet rewarding when coupled with calmness and relaxation through focused breathing. Although challenging, the more effort you invest, the greater the benefits you discover. Maintaining the well-being of your body, including your immune system, through daily focus is essential.

Healing from cancer can take various paths, emphasising the importance of addressing the mind, body and spirit. It is crucial to explore approaches that are most comfortable and suitable for your individual needs.

Daily, Sustainable Approach - *Mind, Body & Spirit*

- De-stress:[4] meditation, positivity, hope, gratitude, connection with family and friends, laugh. Stimulate your Vagus Nerve (refer page 108). Seek out things that bring you joy in your life and continue doing them!

- Move/Exercise:[5] walk, yoga. Even a gentle walk outside will help. Drink lots of filtered water while exercising.

- Nutrition:[7-8] natural pre & probiotics, supplements, reduce carbs, sugar and animal protein, feed the microbiome. Eat a large variety of fruits and vegetables.

- Intravenous Vitamin C:[9-10] A potent antioxidant and immune system enhancer, it is particularly effective when the immune system is fully functional - meaning, it is most effective when used before undergoing any treatments such as chemotherapy. Intravenous Vitamin C - administered periodically

- Release suppressed emotions[6], increase positive emotions (you may need assistance from a professional)

- When able... Run/Weights/High Intensity Interval Training HIIT (2-3 times per week). Brief, intense exercise is incredibly beneficial![11]

- Connect with nature[12], breathe deeply... and repeat

- Feed your soul through prayer or by doing things of a spiritual nature.[13] Focus on helping others.

Combining exercise with a mindful, meditative approach gives you a complete mind-body workout. Various forms of yoga provide this perfect mind body spirit balance.

Intermittent fasting[14] and Fecal Microbiota Transplant (FMT)[15] are powerful emerging anticancer approaches.

Get more sleep!

Forgive yourself & others, practice gratitude

EAT HEALTHY
Salads, juices, veggies, nuts, seeds, Vit C

EXERCISE
Walk, yoga, run, when able... HIIT 2-3 times per wk

TODAY
Choose Healthy

Tomorrow
REPEAT!

Feed your soul, pray, help others

Spend time with family. Walk dog!

Speak to friends & loved ones

DE-STRESS
Breathe, meditate, release supressed emotion, sing

Increase positive emotions

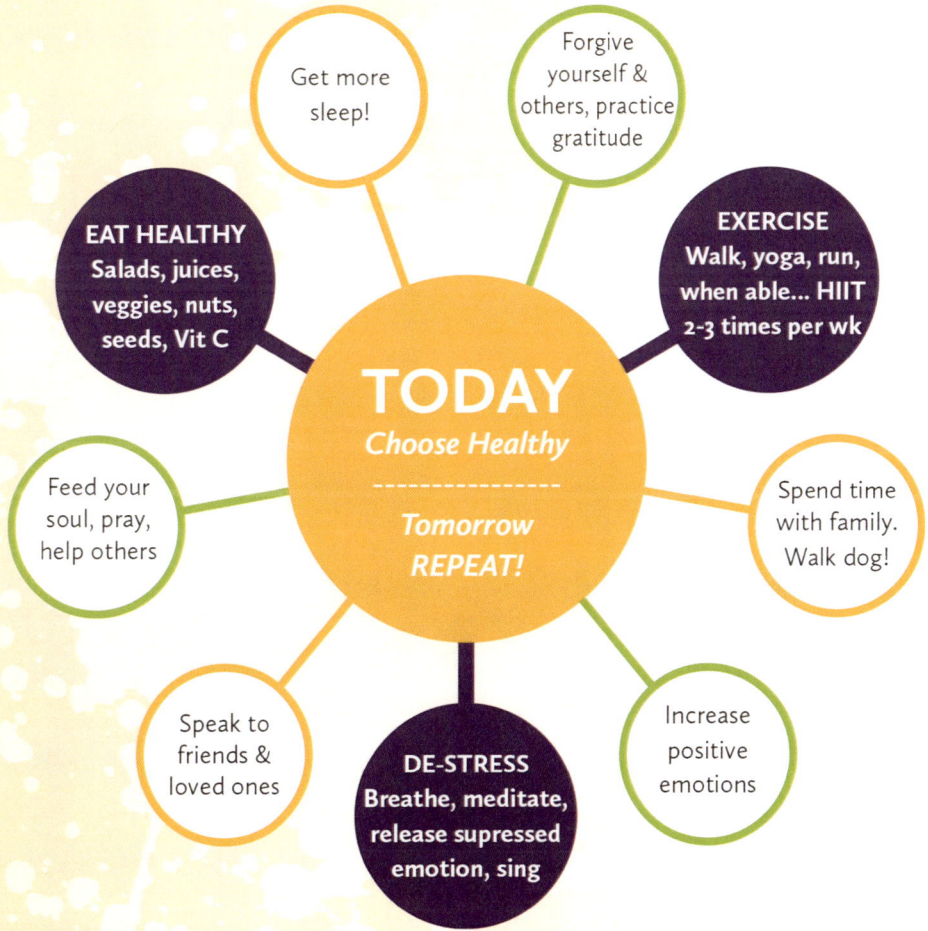

May be combined with or supported by:

Intravenous Vitamin C
Fecal Microbiota Transplant
Intermittent fasting

Natural /Holistic Approach
Mind ~ Body ~ Spirit
Balanced Microbiome and Strong Immune System

Exercise
Walk, Yoga, Stimulate Vagus Nerve, Cycle, Swim, Spend time in nature, When able... Short, intense exercise everyday, Run, HIIT.

HEAL

Nutrition
Fruit & veggies, Pre & Probiotics, Fasting, Intravenous Vitamin C, Supplements

Wellbeing
Meditation, Pray, Mindfulness, Gratitude, Sleep, Laugh, Spiritual & Emotional Healing

May be combined with or supported by:

Fecal Microbiota Transplant

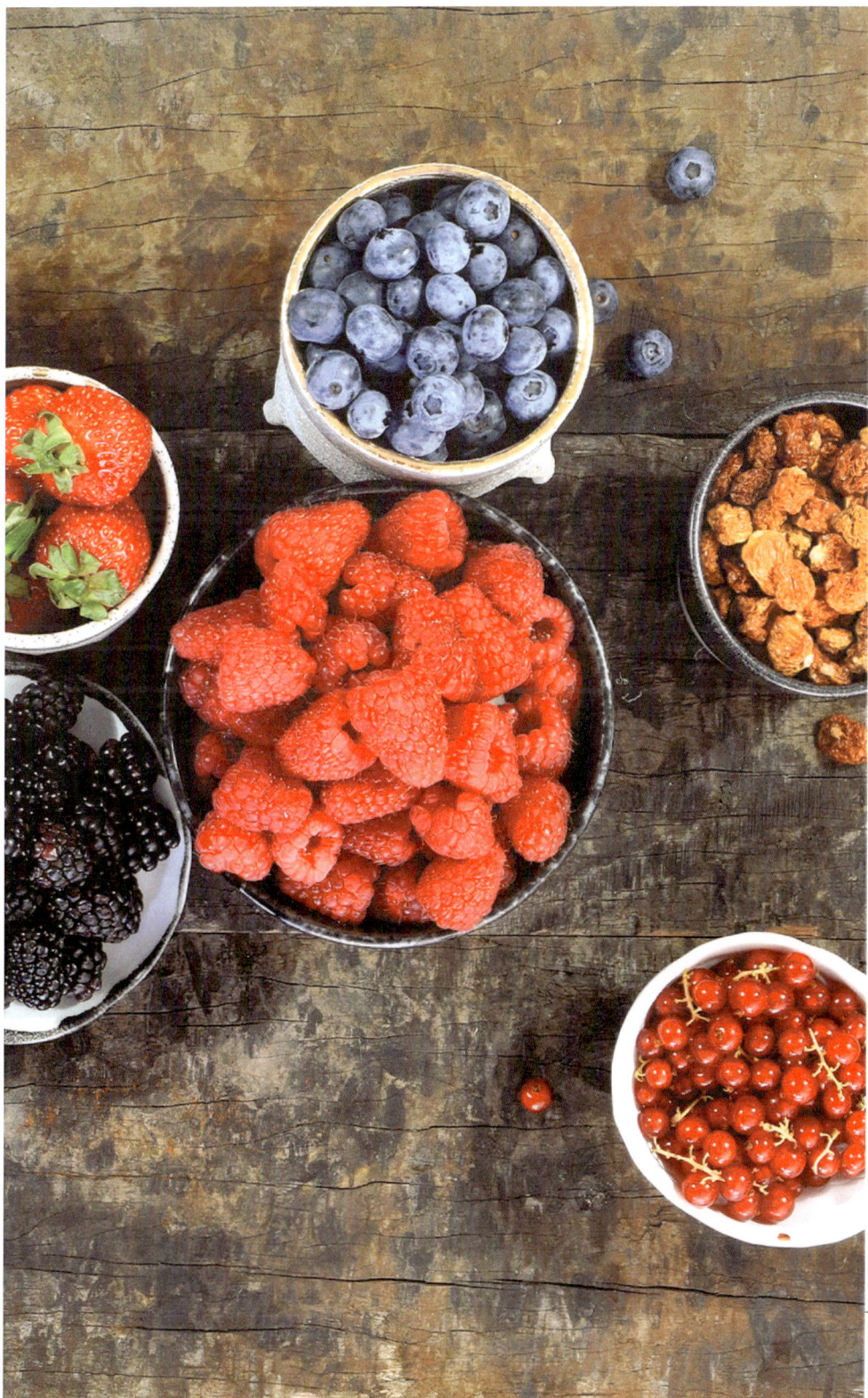

CANCER

Cancer is a disease of the cells in our body. Each cell contains mitochondria that create energy from glucose in an oxidative process called metabolism. Healthy cells grow, get worn out and die in a normal renewal process. Cancer cells are damaged or abnormal cells that create energy through the non-oxidative process of fermentation. There are many types of cancer and it can start in any part of the body. At any given time we may have cancer cells floating throughout our bodies but a healthy system seeks out and destroys them before they can cause problems.

When the immune system isn't functioning correctly these cancer cells aren't all destroyed and continue to grow and replicate. This can lead to single or multiple tumours that develop their own blood vessels through angiogenesis. Cancer cells may break off and spread throughout the body via the blood or lymph vessels. Cancer rates are increasing worldwide.

One in two men and one in three women will be diagnosed with cancer in their lifetime.[1]

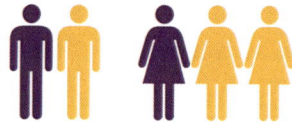

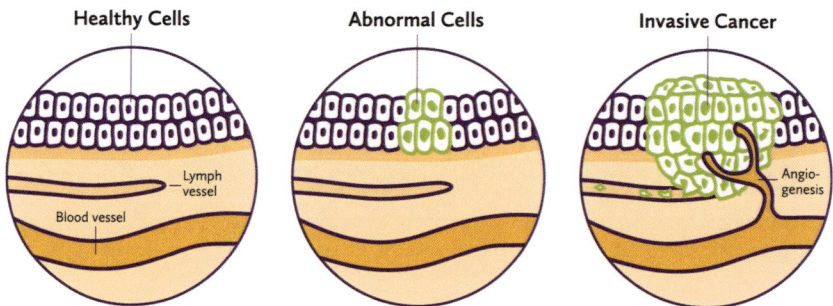

Healthy Cells	Abnormal Cells	Invasive Cancer

Healthy Cells — Lymph vessel, Blood vessel

Invasive Cancer — Angiogenesis

What Causes Cancer

Cancer is a complex group of more than 100 different diseases. Most are caused by unhealthy diets and lifestyles[2] and extremely stressful events.[3] Stress causes inflammation, reduces the immune system's effectiveness and adaptability, and has been clearly linked to disease. Most of us have an understanding of what is and isn't healthy. Smoking, eating highly processed foods, lack of exercise, extreme stress, serious long term sleep problems, sun damage and exposure to environmental toxins can all lead to health issues. Residues of environmental toxins can be found in our foods and products. Our foods are produced using highly toxic pesticides and herbicides such as Glyphosate (Roundup), antibiotics and hormones.

Emotional trauma can create embedded stress in our bodies which may lead to cancer. Often cancer patients can point to a significantly stressful event six months to two years before their cancer diagnosis. Some types of cancer are linked to family genetics. We can alter the way our bodies read our genes by modifying our diets and lifestyles. This is called epigenetics ('in addition to' our standard gene function). Cancer is unique to the individual and tumours change over time which may also be why the immune system may struggle to cope with it.

Standard Treatments

Common cancer treatments include surgery, chemotherapy, radiation therapy, immunotherapy, targeted therapy, hormone therapy, stem cell transplant and precision medicine.

A Holistic Approach

Holistic refers to a mind, body, and spirit approach that considers many of the natural interrelated body systems. It focusses on ways the body maintains health. These can include exercise, adopting a healthy diet and lifestyle, releasing suppressed emotions, improving the gut microbiome, stimulating the vagus nerve, eating organic foods, using filtered water, reducing stress, increasing positive emotions, reducing negative ones, improving sleep, meditation, and yoga, supplements and reducing exposure to environmental toxins. Intermittent fasting has been shown to lengthen life, reduce disease and contribute to overall health[4].

A catalyst for CHANGE

Sometimes a crisis or change is forced upon us. If you've been diagnosed with cancer it can feel like your whole world has been turned upside down. Fear of the unknown and what the future holds, lots of medical appointments and an overload of information creates a great deal of stress and anxiety. You are exhausted! You don't need to panic. Breathe, slow down and think deeply about your situation.
In many cases, your body has allowed cancer to form over time. That can be reversed, you can manage the cancer and/or heal... over time. Many cancers result from unhealthy diets, poor lifestyle choices, extremely stressful events and lack of exercise. Managing and/or healing your cancer won't be easy. It will require you to be focussed, active and empowered to make changes in your life. "If you keep doing what you've always done, you'll keep getting what you've always got." T. Harv Eker.

Never too old, never too bad, never too late, never too sick to start from scratch once again.

Bikram Choudhury

What can help motivate you to make and keep going with changes?

- The fear of cancer and the will to live can serve as crucial initial motivators for change. However, joy and positive reinforcement are more significant for sustaining lasting changes.

- Love and support from your family and friends can inspire healthier choices and help you maintain those choices.

- Hope for remission or cure can encourage you to adopt healthier habits.

- Improving diet and exercise can enhance your overall quality of life during and after cancer treatment.

- Taking control of aspects like diet and exercise can empower you during a challenging time.

- Learning from others' experiences and understanding the link between lifestyle and cancer can be a strong motivator for positive changes.

Embrace Change ~ New Possibilities

Empower yourself and realise you can steer and take charge of the situation. You are adaptable. You are resilient. You are bold.

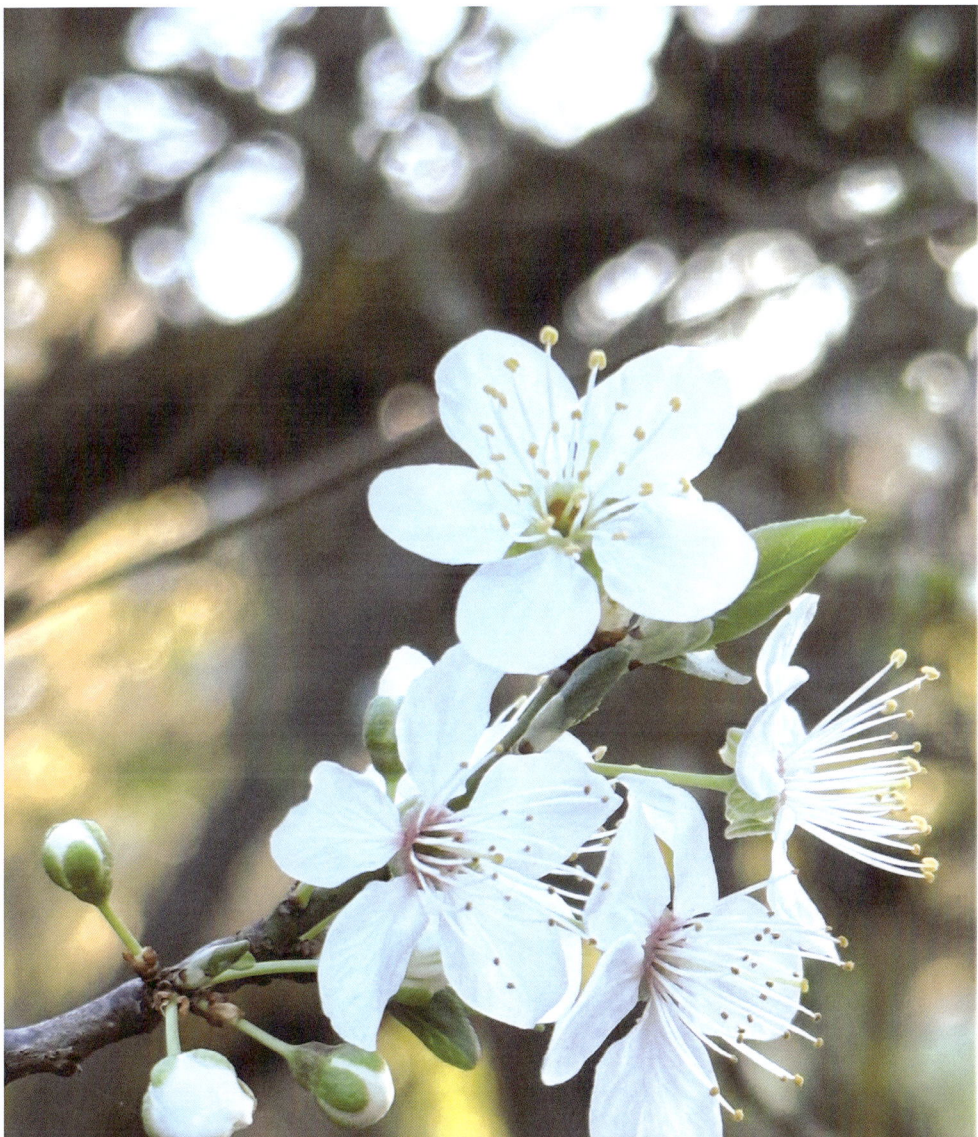

Your life does not get better by chance,
it gets better by change

Jim Rohn

Progress is impossible without change,
and those who cannot change their minds
cannot change anything

George Bernard Shaw

Fear and Stress Paralyses

It's human nature to be scared of the unknown. Fear keeps us from taking excessive risks and potentially harming ourselves in the process. In the past it was an essential emotion to help keep us safe from the wild beasts outside of our campfire light. Fear is a driving force and if it's left unchecked it can overwhelm and wreak havoc. We can overcome anxiety and stress by doing a few different scary things and gradually building our confidence about our ability to manage. Now is the time to be adventurous and try some new/different/challenging things; join a public speaking group or choir, try skydiving or scuba diving, learn a musical instrument. It's not the time to wrap yourself in cotton wool. Your choices are endless. There are so many different things that can challenge you and help you realise it's ok to be scared and that you can manage your fears.

A Healthy Change

You can rebalance and beat this cancer by doing all of the right things to help your body heal. You'll find information in other chapters about mind, body, spirit approaches, releasing suppressed emotions, healthy nutrition, exercise and lifestyle choices that will help you succeed.

Hope

Having hope for a better future helps you cope with your current prognosis. It helps you envision a positive outcome and enables you to take steps to make it happen. You can be reassured you're not on this journey on your own. There are many others who, just like you, have faced this and slowly improved their health to the point where either their cancer is managed or it has gone.

Kelly Turner Ph.D., researched over 1,000 medically documented unexpected remissions (called 'spontaneous remissions' by the medical system) and interviewed survivors and healers. She found that survivors worked hard to improve their health and kept chipping away, making changes until they found what worked for them. Kelly refers to these remissions as 'radical remissions'.

Many of these are detailed in her book 'Radical Hope[1]' and on her website: radicalremission.com

You can heal

SUSTAINABLE CHANGES
Setting and Achieving Goals

Creating ongoing lifestyle and healthier changes requires planning, commitment, gradual adjustments and finding ways to enjoy life along the way. Here's a step-by-step guide to help you make sustainable changes. *You've got this!*

Set Clear Goals

Define Specific, Measurable, Achievable, Relevant, and Time-based (SMART) goals. For example, instead of saying 'I want to be healthier,' set a goal like 'I will exercise for 30 minutes, five days a week, and eat at least five servings of vegetables daily.'

Start Small

Avoid overwhelming yourself by making too many changes at once. Begin with one or two manageable changes, such as incorporating a morning walk or swapping sugary snacks for fruits, nuts or seeds.

Focus on Habits

Concentrate on building healthy habits rather than relying solely on willpower. Habits become automatic over time, making it easier to sustain your efforts.

Create a Routine

Establish a consistent daily routine that includes your healthier choices. This routine will make it easier to stick to your goals and minimise decision fatigue.

Enjoy the Journey

Make sure you find ways to enjoy what you're doing to keep the momentum going! That might include practicing gratitude or concentrating on aspects of your goals that truly make you happy.

Track Progress

Keep a journal or use a tracking app to monitor your progress. Recording your achievements can provide motivation and help you identify areas that may need adjustment.

Stay Accountable

Share your goals with a friend, family member, or join a supportive community. Accountability partners can provide encouragement and celebrate your successes with you.

Gradual Changes

Slowly incorporate changes to give your body and mind time to adjust. This reduces the chances of feeling overwhelmed and increases the likelihood of long-term success.

Nutrition

Focus on a diet rich in fruits, vegetables, lean proteins, whole grains, and healthy fats. Opt for sustainable eating patterns.

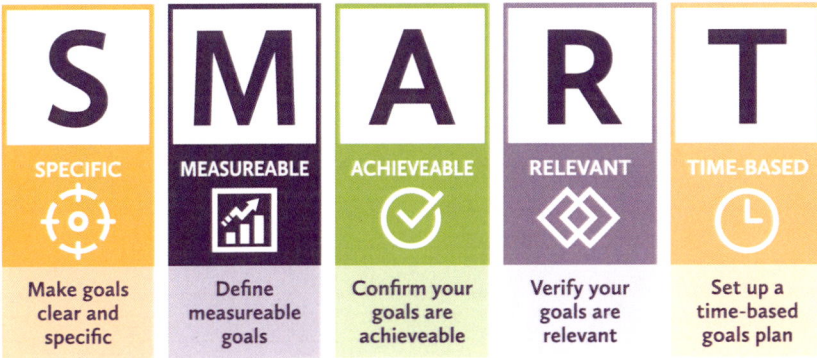

S	M	A	R	T
SPECIFIC	**MEASUREABLE**	**ACHIEVEABLE**	**RELEVANT**	**TIME-BASED**
Make goals clear and specific	Define measureable goals	Confirm your goals are achieveable	Verify your goals are relevant	Set up a time-based goals plan

Physical Activity

Engage in regular physical activity you enjoy. Whether it's walking, swimming, dancing, weightlifting, etc. Consistency is key. Aim for at least 150 minutes of moderate-intensity aerobic activity per week, at least three sessions of short high intensity activities, along with muscle-strengthening exercises.

Sleep and Stress Management

Prioritise sleep and manage stress through techniques like meditation, deep breathing, yoga, or spending time in nature. Adequate sleep and stress reduction are vital for overall health.

Hydration

Drink plenty of water throughout the day. Staying hydrated supports various bodily functions and can help with appetite control.

Mindful Eating

Pay attention to your body's hunger and fullness cues. Eat slowly, savor your food, and avoid distractions like screens during meals.

Celebrate Milestones

Celebrate your achievements along the way, whether it's completing a month of eating healthy foods or consistent exercise. The best rewards are not related to food and might include going to a movie with a friend. Rewarding yourself reinforces positive behavior.

Adapt and Learn

Be open to adjusting your plan as needed. Life can be unpredictable, so flexibility is important for maintaining your healthy lifestyle in different situations.

Long-Term Perspective

Remember that creating lasting changes takes time. Focus on the journey and the positive impacts on your overall well-being rather than quick fixes.

By following these steps and maintaining a patient and positive attitude, you can gradually incorporate healthier habits into your daily life and **create sustainable lifestyle changes**. *Enjoy!*

CANCER *Managers & Survivors*

Dr Nasha Winters ND FABNO

In 1991, Nasha was diagnosed with end-stage ovarian cancer and given 3-6 months to live. Because of the advanced stage of the disease and overt organ failure she was sent to palliative care. She has since embarked on a nearly 30 year journey exploring all parts of her mind, body, spirit, diet and lifestyle and adjusted anything that needed attention being determined not to be another statistic. She graduated from Naturopathic Medical school and Acupuncture school and spent countless hours mentoring and shadowing physicians in every field worldwide. She has been cancer stable for nearly two decades now. Nasha has found that seemingly healthy people who develop cancer have underlying conditions or terrain that have contributed to their diagnosis and has developed a range of questionnaires to assess potential problem areas. Her focus is then on creating the most suitable food and changes to enhance healing. She continues to share her story consulting with physicians worldwide and works hard to effect real change in the global understanding and treatment of cancer. She is currently focused on opening a comprehensive metabolic oncology hospital and research institute in the US which will offer the most advanced integrative therapies.

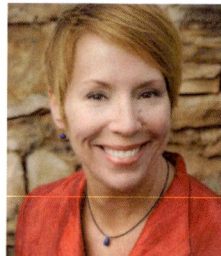

Book: The Metabolic Approach to Cancer   **drnasha.com**

Ted Howard

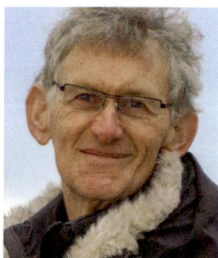

Ted had stage 4 metastatic malignant melanoma. He was diagnosed in 2008 and cancer free in 2011. After multiple surgeries he was told he was beyond medical help and might only have six weeks to live. He was offered palliative care and sent home. He focussed on a vegan, half raw diet, daily doses of Vitamin C (minimum of two heaped teaspoons pure L Ascorbic acid per day dissolved in a glass of luke warm water), multiple vitamins, no added sugar and remains reasonably active. Ted continues to live a healthy life.

tedhowardnz.wordpress.com/about

Di Foster

"You have secondary terminal breast cancer, metastasised in your lungs; your life expectancy is 12 months, no chance of 18months, go home and pop your affairs in order." It was 2010, and I was 38 years old. I had a choice to make. I could spend the next year fighting and doing treatment that was not life-extending, or I could listen to my own heart. You see, I had heard the whispers - Be Present - Go Natural - Be Grateful. That was 11 years ago. I survived to tell the story and if telling my story helps one person, then today is a good day. The goal was not to heal. The very best I could wish for was to reduce my symptoms and maybe get five years. I reduced my symptoms so much, I healed. I'm continuing to embrace natural approaches and I'm thriving, being present and grateful. Much gratitude, DI x

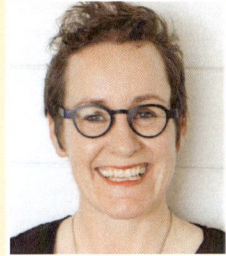

difoster.com

Chris Wark

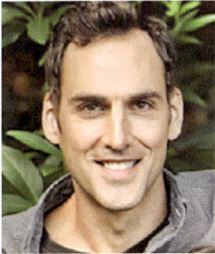

In December 2003 I was diagnosed with Stage IIIc colon cancer. There was a golf ball sized tumor in my large intestine, and the cancer had spread to my lymph nodes. It was two days before Christmas, and I was 26 years old. The oncologist told me I was "insane" but I decided against chemotherapy after surgery. After prayerful consideration I radically changed my diet and did every natural non-toxic therapy I could find. Seven years later, in 2010, I started this blog to share my story and everything I've learned about nutrition and natural cancer therapies. I also started sharing cancer healing testimonials from other survivors. Fast forward to 2021... By the grace of God, I'm still cancer-free, healthy and strong, and in the best shape of my life. My wife and I have two beautiful daughters, Marin and Mackenzie. I thank Him every day for my life, health and healing.

Book: Chris Beat Cancer   chrisbeatcancer.com
'Square One' Coaching Program

Glenn Sabin

Glenn had advanced, incurable, Chronic Lymphocytic Leukemia. Diagnosed in 1991 and cancer-free in 2012, he attributes his healing without conventional treatment correlated to his commitment to a plant-strong diet, well-placed supplements, stress reduction techniques, social connection, filtered water and quality sleep. He believes the brain is the most powerful and least understood organ in the human body - and that the healing of any disease starts with a calm unfettered mind and strong will to live. Glenn believes that healing takes many forms and even though he achieved his ultimate healing without conventional treatment he still sees the importance of conventional care, augmented by natural, lifestyle-driven approaches. He is not only surviving but thriving.

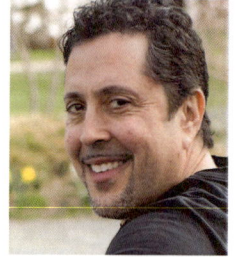

Book: 'n of 1' **glennsabin.com**

Ryan Sternagel (Father of Ryder)

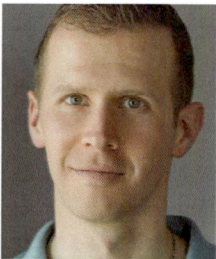

Imagine this... On your son or daughter's 1st birthday, they are diagnosed with cancer. What do you do? Well, this horrifying event actually happened to Ryan & Teddy Sternagel's son, Ryder in 2014. At age one, Ryder was diagnosed with neuroblastoma. Ryan and wife Teddy, consulted countless doctors and health experts of all disciplines to employ an integrative approach that cut the amount of conventional treatment Ryder received in half through an integrative mix of super nutrition, complementary therapies and energy medicine, along with a whole lot of prayer and healthy lifestyle changes. Today Ryder is thriving and enjoying life like never before! Ryan and Teddy are now the founders of 'The Stern Method', a platform helping other families.

Book: 'The Ultimate Healthy Home Checklist'
thesternmethod.com

Jenny Kennedy

In 2012 Jenny was diagnosed with Stage 3C ovarian cancer. After having been told by the medical profession that they could not cure her she set about following her intuitive guidance to heal herself. This involved eating healthily, dancing, doing Qi Gong, swimming, massage, supplements, walking in fresh air and most importantly getting to the root cause of what created the cancer by uncovering events in the past where she had experienced trauma and suppressed emotion. She is thrilled to say that she is now healthy and, according to her oncologist, "as far as I am concerned you are free of cancer".

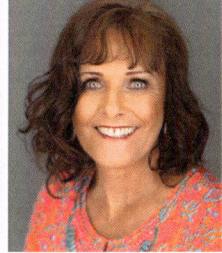

jennykennedy.co.nz

Cathy Brown

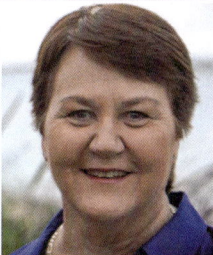

In 1990 Cathy was diagnosed with metastatic melanoma and told she had two months to two years to live. Chemo and radiotherapy were not an option, so she had to find another way to heal as her children were only six and eight years old. This led her on an incredible healing journey over many years. She followed a strict naturopathic diet, focussed on alternative healing approaches most importantly controlling her mind through meditation, energy healing, acupuncture, reiki, kinesiology and found great comfort in a Cancer Support Group. Several check-ups later, 22 months after having the secondary tumors removed from under my arm, the Oncologist informed her that he didn't need to see her anymore. That was in 1992 and since then she has gone on to write a book of her story, has set up her own business LifeXL and continues to inspire and support many others. She is currently working with Dr Ian Gawler on a pilot program helping people use his 'Allevi8' app (allevi8.net) which helps people train their mind into stillness instead of stress and anxiety.

Book: My Answer to Cancer   lifexl.com.au

Dr Ian Gawler OAM

In 1975 Ian, a 24 year old veterinarian developed bone cancer and his right leg was amputated. The cancer returned and in 1976 he was given weeks to live. Ian embarked upon an holistic health regime focusing on anticancer nutrition, a positive attitude, regular intense meditation and the acceptance of loving support. Later, he had palliative radiotherapy and some experimental chemotherapy. In 1978 he was declared cancer-free. In 1981 Ian founded the Gawler Foundation. One of the pioneers in Body/Mind Medicine, Ian has spoken at many conferences and seminars worldwide on topics such as overcoming cancer, eating for recovery, meditation and inner peace. Currently Ian is engaged with developing a mindfulness and meditation app specifically designed for people affected by chronic degenerative diseases including cancer, a meditation retreat for young people and a Centre for Contemplative Studies at a major Melbourne University.

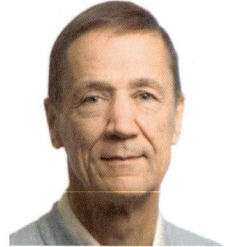

Books include: You Can Conquer Cancer and Blue Sky Mind
App: Allevi8   iangawler.com

Sara Hamo

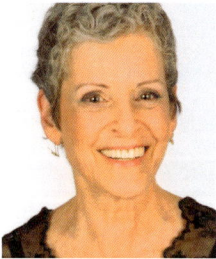

At the age of 34 in 1979 Sara was diagnosed with a Stage 4 Non-Hodgkin's Lymphoma. She started chemo but was very distressed and searched for a more balanced and natural healing method. She found the Kingston method that relies on an improved diet, a good night's sleep at the right hours and a more robust approach to healthy activities such as walking. Medicine makes us dependent, freeing us from our own health responsibility. She passionately believes we must acknowledge our ignorance and so unleash the body's power for self-healing through a pure and balanced nutrition. She has helped thousands of people in her clinic.

Book: The Golden Path to Natural Healing   naturalway.co.il

You can also find many more survivor stories on Kelly Turner's Radical Remission website: **radicalremission.com**

Justine Laidlaw

In 2013 Justine was 45 years old and was diagnosed with a Stage 3 aggressive colon cancer. After trying to detox without early success she chose surgical treatment. Following surgery her prognosis with or without chemo or radiation was dire. She chose integrative and holistic options instead believing that her body had created this tumour and a poisonous approach wasn't going to fix it. She focussed on the needs of her body, mind and soul and made daily adjustments. She maintained strong reasons for living, released fear-based emotions, worked with a holistic clinic, underwent ozone therapy, overhauled her food choices, used herbs and supplements and essential oils and focussed on her mental, emotional and spiritual needs. Six months after her surgery a scan showed she had one enlarged cancerous lymph node. She trusted in her intuition and monitored subsequent scans and was declared 'NED' (No evidence of Disease) in 2015.

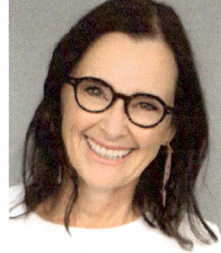

thenaturalbird.co.nz

Anita Moorjani

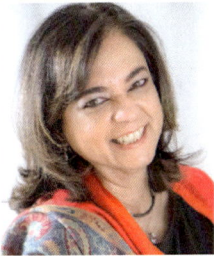

In 2002 Anita was diagnosed with a stage 2 lymphoma (cancer of the lymphatic system). She chose to focus solely on holistic therapies but after four years her cancer had progressed to the point where she finally accepted chemotherapy, but doctors told her it was too late to save her. She slipped into a coma in hospital. During the coma she had a near death experience (NDE) where she realised she was overly fearful and that this was undermining her health efforts. She felt she had become unwell because she had been suppressing her emotions, harshly treating and judging herself and pleasing everyone rather than being true to herself. At that point during the NDE instead of letting go she chose to come back. With a dramatically different approach she was completely healed within six months. Multiple oncologists have verified her story.

Books include: Dying to Be Me, Sensitive is The New Strong
anitamoorjani.com

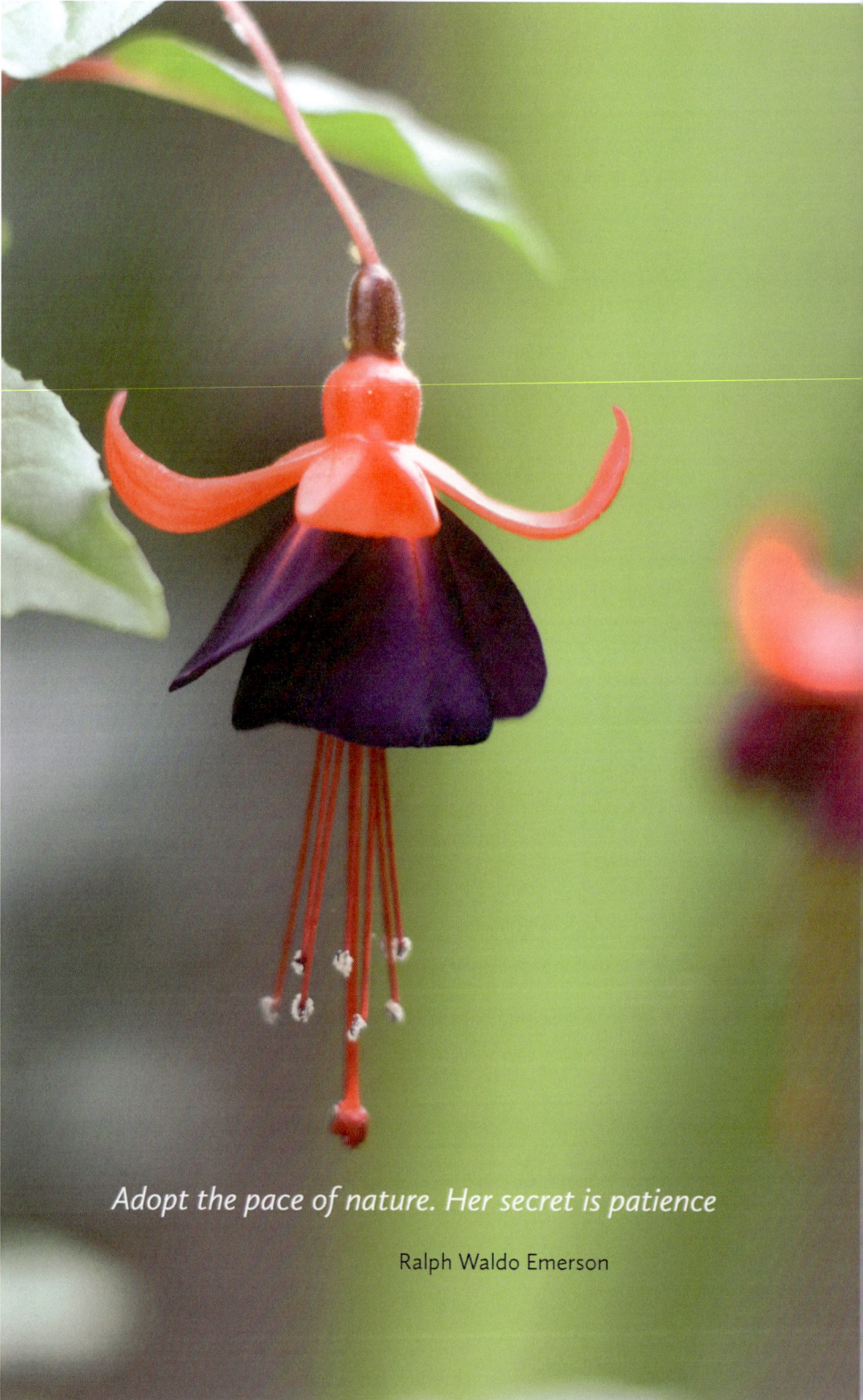

Adopt the pace of nature. Her secret is patience

Ralph Waldo Emerson

BRAIN-GUT
Communication

The digestive system or gut includes the mouth, esophagus, stomach, pancreas, liver, gallbladder and small and large intestines. The large intestine (cecum, colon, rectum, and anal canal) contains a massive community of trillions of microorganisms including bacteria, fungi and viruses. There are **four times more** of these cells compared to our human cells. The gut has a large surface area and comes into contact with a significant amount of food. It is also called the 'second brain' because it contains a large number of neurotransmitters and is in constant communication with the brain[1]. It has more neurons than the spinal column.

The gut microbiome manages 70% of your immune system[2] and can affect mood, behaviour and neurological functioning. Poor food and lifestyle choices can create a great deal of inflammation in the gut significantly affecting health. Medications, including antibiotics, have been shown to reduce the gut microbiome's good flora.[3-4] Eating a large variety of prebiotics (foods that contain lots of fibre such as fruits and vegetables) and probiotics (food and drink that contains live, good bacteria) will feed the good bacteria and help ensure your gut is healthy. Regular and intense exercise is also a key factor. Keep well hydrated with lots of filtered water to aid digestion and maintain a healthy microbiome. Periodic fasting allows the digestive system to rest and repair damage and inflammation, which is essential for long term health. When there is severe gut malfunction, a fecal microbiota transplant (FMT) can restore gut bacteria's healthy balance. Emerging research indicates strong links between gut flora and cancer outcomes.[5] The FMT works by transferring a processed mixture of liquid poo from a healthy donor into the patient's intestines restoring the healthy gut bacteria.

Keeping the Gut Healthy

- Microbiome contains bacteria, fungi and viruses and manages 70% of the immune system

- Affects mood, behaviour and brain function

- Eat a large variety of prebiotic foods (containing fibre) such as fruits and vegetables. Eat and drink probiotics foods (live, good bacteria)

- Regular, intense exercise and drinking lots of filtered water is key

- Periodic fasting, rests and repairs the gut

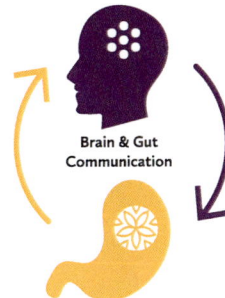

Brain & Gut Communication

THE IMMUNE SYSTEM

The immune system is a vast network of cells, tissues and organs that protects the body from harmful substances, damaged cells and disease. It's made up of white blood cells, antibodies, the complement system, the lymphatic system, tonsils, spleen, thymus, appendix and bone marrow. If a pathogen or damaging substance gets into our bodies, the immune system produces white blood cells and other chemicals and proteins to attack and destroy it. It learns and remembers the attack and launches a quick response when attacked again by the same substance.

How to Keep it Healthy

- Eat a large variety of fruits and vegetables. Ideally 20-30 different sorts each week

- Exercise regularly and drink a lot of filtered water

- If you drink alcohol, drink only in moderation

- Get adequate sleep

- Take steps to avoid infection, such as washing your hands frequently and cooking meats thoroughly

- Try to minimise stress. Laugh, a lot.

- Stimulate the Vagus Nerve (refer pg 84)

Walking is an easy way to build and strengthen your immune system. A simple 10-minute walk brings a lot of health benefits. For best results, increase to a fast-paced walk, 45 minutes per day to achieve a meditative state.

The Immune System and Cancer

Cancer cells are formed from the patients own DNA and so the immune system may not always recognise it as a threat or foreign invader.[1] A weakened or stressed immune system may struggle to keep up with fast-growing cancer cells. The best advice is to keep your immune system as healthy as possible.[2]

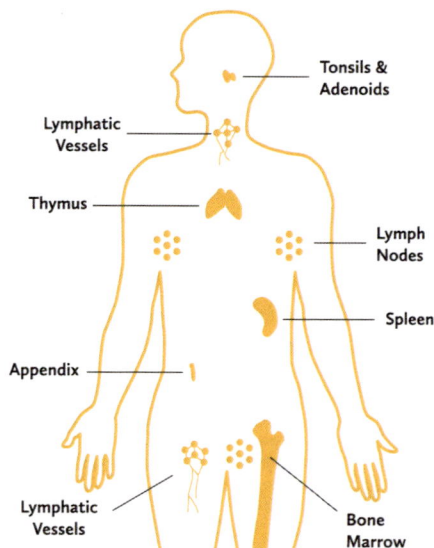

Tonsils & Adenoids
Lymphatic Vessels
Thymus
Lymph Nodes
Spleen
Appendix
Lymphatic Vessels
Bone Marrow

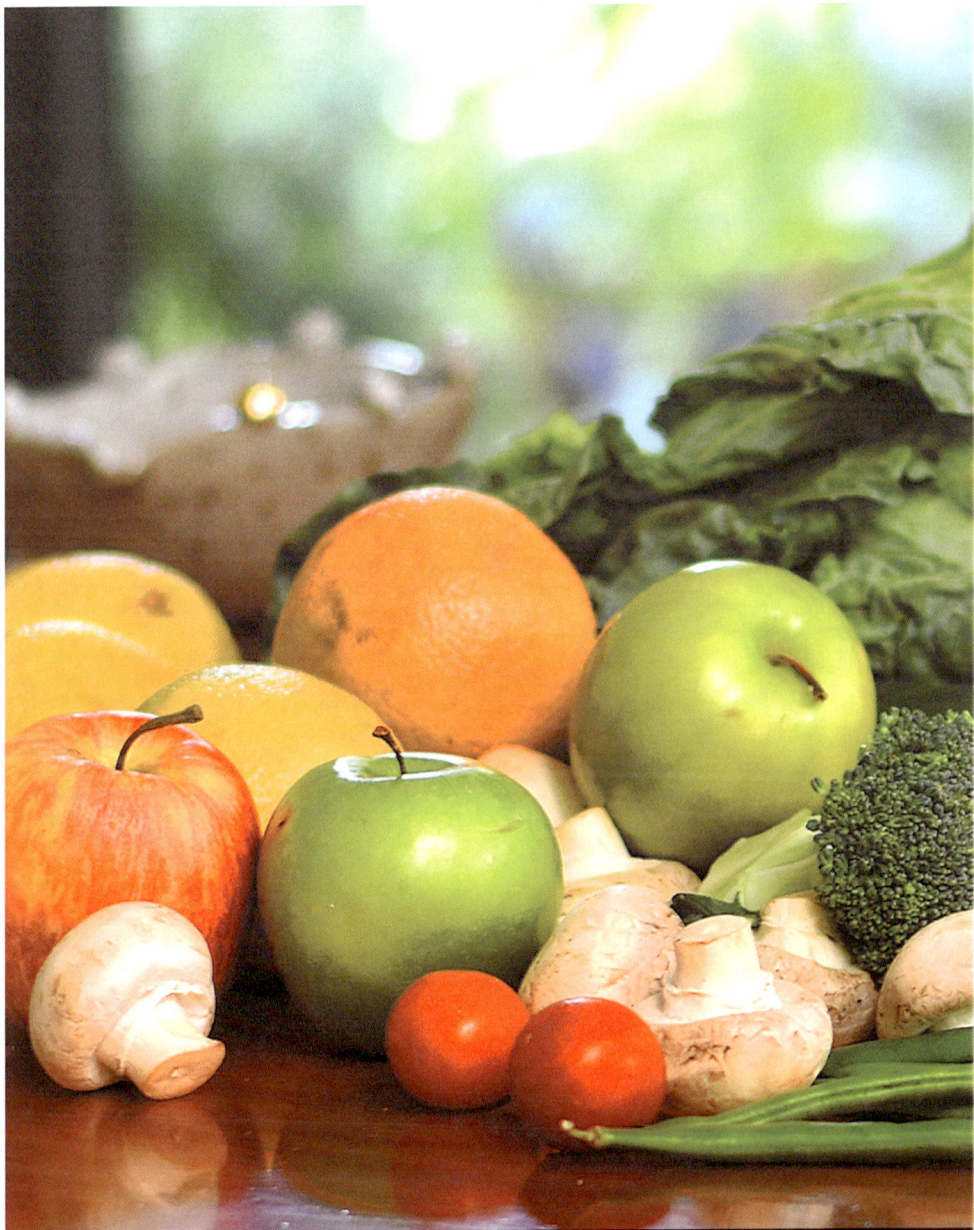

If you want to have a healthy immune system, you need to laugh often, view life with a positive eye, and put yourself in a relaxed state of mind on a regular basis

Michael T. Murray

EXERCISE

"Cancer patients who exercise regularly experience fewer and less severe side effects from treatments. They also have a lower relative risk of cancer recurrence and a lower relative risk of dying from their cancer." Prue Cormie[1-2] is part of Australia's peak body representing health professionals who treat people with cancer, the Clinical Oncology Society of Australia (COSA).

Cancer patients have traditionally been told to rest and avoid activity but substantial research has found exercise does reduce the side effects of chemo or radiation and also contributes to keeping cancer under control. COSA recommends "...all health professionals involved in the care of people with cancer should:[3-4]

- View and discuss exercise as a standard part of the cancer treatment plan

- Recommend people with cancer adhere to exercise guidelines

- Refer patients to an exercise physiologist or physiotherapist with experience in cancer care"

Prue says "If the effects of exercise could be encapsulated in a pill, it would be prescribed to every cancer patient worldwide and viewed as a major breakthrough in cancer treatment."

She goes on to say, "Research shows exercise can help cancer patients tolerate aggressive treatments, minimise the physical declines caused by cancer, counteract cancer-related fatigue, relieve mental distress and improve quality of life. When appropriately prescribed and monitored, exercise is safe for people with cancer and the risk of complications is relatively low."

The Best Exercise for you ~ *DAILY*

- Walk fast-paced 45 minutes per day, breathe deeply and connect with nature. Drink lots of filtered water

- Yoga / meditation / release suppressed emotions / increase positive emotions / practice gratitude

- When able... Run/Swim/High Intensity Interval Training HIIT (2-3 times per week)

- Weight-bearing gym work (supervised... to ensure it's appropriate to your needs) 2-3 times per week

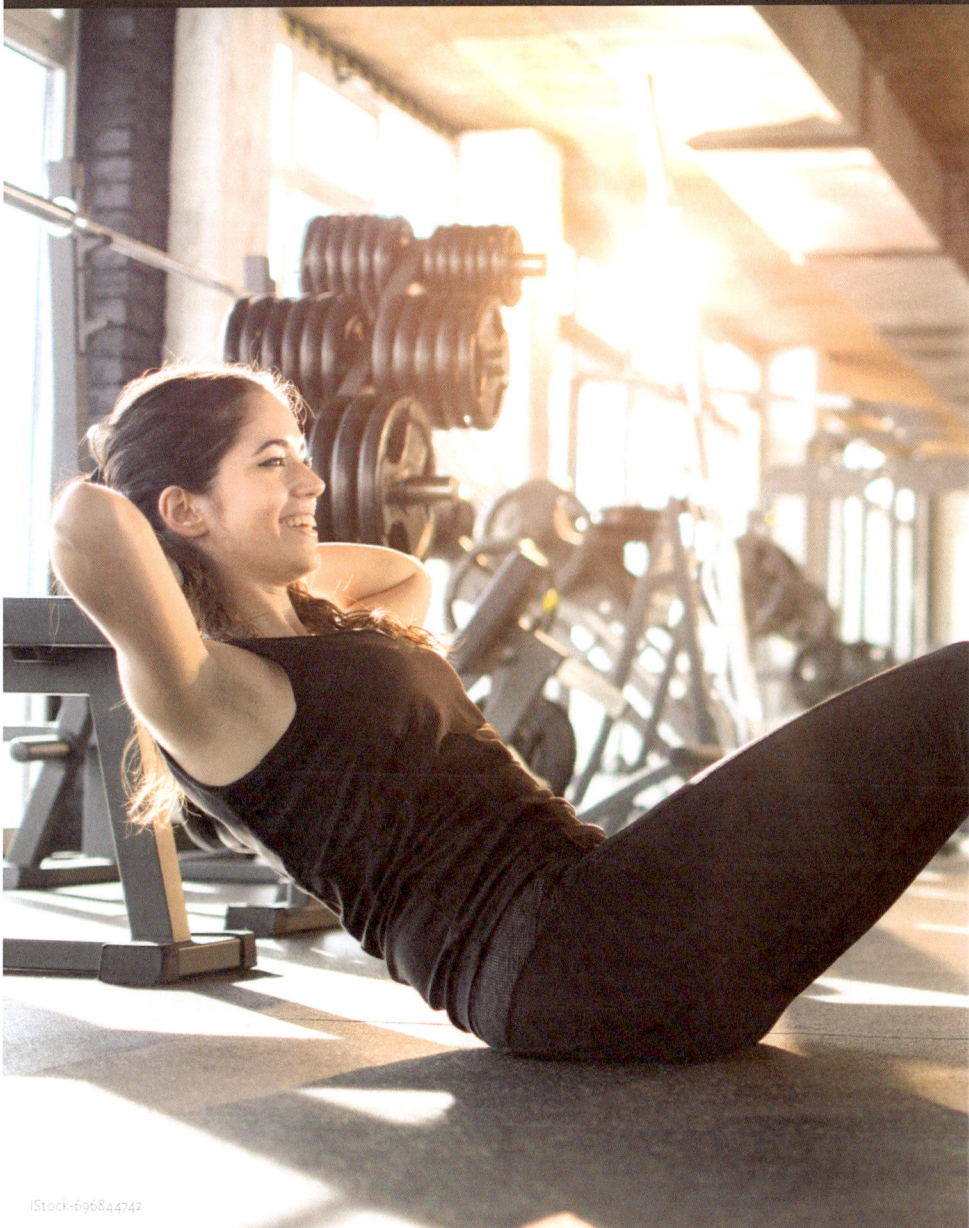

> *Only one in ten will exercise enough during and after their [cancer] treatment but every one of them would greatly benefit from exercise*
>
> Prue Cormie, Clinical Oncology Society of Australia (COSA)

NUTRITION
Choose Organic Where Possible

Quality, organic nutrition in conjunction with daily exercise and lifestyle changes reducing stress will enable your immune system to perform at its peak and may reduce and heal cancer over time.[1-2]

Four cellular processes have been linked to either controlling or promoting cancer growth. These include inflammation, oxidative stress, blood sugar regulation/insulin production and normal cell death (apoptosis). If these processes are out of balance the immune system can become stressed and overwhelmed and cancer can proliferate.[3]

> *"The best way to beat back the disease is by creating a healthy biological environment that makes it difficult (or impossible, the best-case scenario) for cancer cells to flourish. The right foods can help accomplish this task."*[3]
>
> Donald I. Abrams, MD, Chief, Hematology-Oncology

The powerhouse of your immune system is your microbiome. Feed it.

Eat a large variety of high fibre foods, in other words an organic plant-rich diet, including lots of vegetables, fruit, nuts, legumes, herbs and spices. Variety is the key. Often we tend to eat the same types of foods and rely on fast foods. This lack of diversity and quality feeds the bacteria that causes inflammation. A high fibre diet ensures the bulk of your food intake moves through to your large intestine where most of your good gut flora lives and works. This will provide the greatest boost to your gut biome and, therefore, to your overall immune system, as a principal component of fighting the symptoms and long-term effects of cancer.

Top of the list are antioxidant-rich, anti-inflammatory wholefoods. Drink plenty of organic green juices and eat lots of salads. Avoid highly processed foods and in particular animal protein, red and processed meats.[4-5]

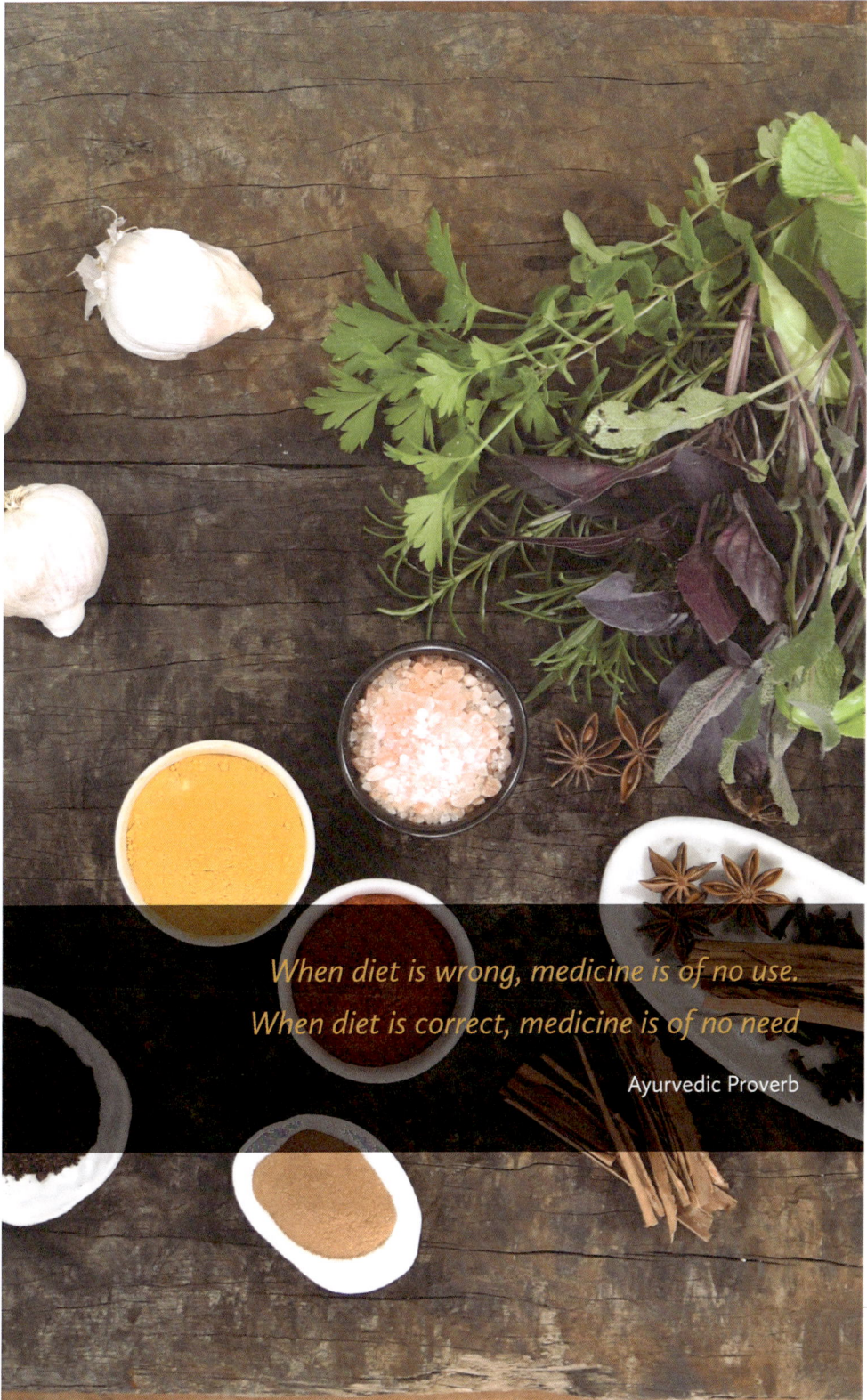

When diet is wrong, medicine is of no use.
When diet is correct, medicine is of no need

Ayurvedic Proverb

Colourful fruits & veggies

Brightly coloured pigments in plant foods indicate high levels of phytochemicals, especially carotenoid antioxidants and Vitamin A. Phytonutrients are chemicals produced by plants that help them grow well and defend themselves from predators and pathogens. When we consume phytonutrients, we take on their benefits as well. These foods include citrus fruits, carrots, apples, sweet potatoes, capsicums, pumpkin, tomatoes, squashes and other plant foods.

Mediterranean Diet

The Mediterranean diet has been shown to combat cancer[1]. It consists of plant-based foods, such as fruits and vegetables, whole grains, legumes and nuts. Replacing butter with healthy fats such as olive oil. Using herbs and spices instead of salt to flavour foods.

Ketogenic Diet

The low carbohydrate or ketogenic diet is a promising and effective anticancer approach.[2-3] Eating a low carb diet switches your cell metabolism to burn fat instead of sugar or glucose. This creates a metabolic state known as ketosis. Cancer cells aren't able to switch their metabolism in the same way normal cells can, so they are starved of their fuel. This may be most effective in the initial stages of fighting cancer. Choose a low protein or vegetarian version of the diet. Over the longer term it's essential to also provide a diverse range of healthy foods for the gut biome to maximise its immune and anti-inflammatory capabilities.

Benefits of juicing

Juicing is an effective way for your body to receive large quantities of vital nutrients for healing. It's essential to continue to eat plant-based foods including fruits, vegetables, nuts, herbs and spices. This ensures your gut biome receives plenty of fibre rather than just a quick hit of nutrients from the juice. Other benefits include hydration, creating alkalinity, reducing inflammation, and eliminating toxins by assisting the liver's cleansing action. The best juicers are the masticating type that slowly grind rather than spinning at high speeds.

Leafy green vegetables and sprouts

Cruciferous vegetables such as cabbage, cauliflower, kale, brussels sprouts, broccoli, bok choy and turnips are extremely high in anticancer phytochemicals and antioxidants including vitamin C and beta-carotene (a type of vitamin A). These have both anti-inflammatory and antibacterial properties, detoxify carcinogens and inhibit tumour cell growth. Sprouted forms of these veggies also pack a powerful punch. In particular, broccoli sprouts have a potent antioxidant called Sulforaphane, which has been shown to have powerful anticancer properties.

Berries

Containing the highest antioxidants available, cranberries, blueberries, raspberries, cherries, strawberries, goji berries, camu camu, amla and blackberries contain Vitamins C and A and gallic acid that is a powerful antifungal/antiviral agent that increases immunity.

Herbs and spices

Many herbs and spices can play a significant role in fighting cancer because of their powerful anticancer properties and immune system boosting compounds. These include turmeric/curcumin, fennel, saffron, cumin, cinnamon, oregano, cayenne pepper/capsicum (chilli peppers), ginger, cloves, raw garlic, thyme, basil, parsley, anise, caraway, fenugreek, mustard and many more. Each has its anticancer qualities.

Turmeric/curcumin[1] is perhaps the most potent of all anti-cancer spices. Curcumin is an anti-inflammatory that stops cancer cells dividing, stops tumours from spreading, stops angiogenesis, causes cancer cells to die. Take with black pepper to increase its bio availability.

Nuts and seeds

Chia seeds, flaxseeds, hemp seeds, sesame seeds, pumpkin seeds and sunflower seeds, walnuts, brazil nuts and almonds provide plenty of nutrients and minerals and have various anticancer properties.

Healthy unrefined oils

Refined vegetable oils, hydrogenated oils and trans fats can damage our immune system and lead to inflammation and disease. When possible use flax oil, extra virgin olive oil, cod oil and coconut oil.

Mushrooms

Over the centuries mushrooms have been recognised as immune-enhancers. Different varieties have particular cancer-fighting properties so it's best to research which are best for your cancer. Reishi, cordyceps, and maitake can improve immune function, fight tumour growth and help with cell regeneration.

Teas

Green tea along with some other teas contain many benefits for health. The tea polyphenols, including the catechins, are thought to be the reason for their strong antioxidant activity. Epigallocatechin-3-gallate (EGCG) and Epicatechin-3-gallate (ECG) have substantial free radical scavenging activity and may protect cells from DNA damage. "Tea polyphenols have also been shown to inhibit tumour cell proliferation and induce apoptosis in laboratory and animal studies. In other laboratory and animal studies, tea catechins have been shown to inhibit angiogenesis and tumor cell invasiveness... [and]...may modulate immune system function."[1]

Prebiotic and probiotic foods

As previously mentioned the immune system is primarily supported and influenced by the gut microbiome which consists of trillions of bacteria and microorganisms. Prebiotics and probiotics help the body in building and maintaining a healthy colony of these microorganisms, which supports the gut and aids digestion. Prebiotics are present in fibre-rich foods, such as fruits, vegetables, and whole grains. Probiotics occur in many fermented foods, including yogurt, sauerkraut, and tempeh. Variety is key to providing the greatest benefit to the good bacteria which support immune health.

Honey

Contains flavonoids, phenolic acids, antioxidants as well as other potent anticancer compounds.[2]

Vitamin C: foods and intravenous therapy

Playing a pivotal role in immune system support, vitamin C significantly contributes to the production and functionality of white blood cells, crucial defenders against infections and illnesses. This highlights the vitamin's importance in fortifying the body's natural defence mechanisms. Additionally, vitamin C is indispensable for collagen synthesis, a vital protein providing structure to connective tissues, skin, blood vessels, and bones. This dual role in immune function and tissue maintenance underscores the vitamin's significance in supporting overall bodily resilience.

A number of foods are high in vitamin C including citrus fruits, berries, tropical fruits, melons, cruciferous veggies (broccoli etc), leafy greens (spinach etc), capsicums, tomatoes, papaya and guava. It's advisable to monitor vitamin C levels during and after treatment to ensure they remain adequate.

Intravenous Vitamin C:
Refer to page 12

Other vitamins and supplements

In most cases sourcing your vitamins and minerals from fresh foods is best. Cancer and other diseases can deplete these resources in the body more rapidly than they can be replenished. This is when it's essential to add supplements into the diet for a while. Fresh is always best in the long term. Selenium removes free radicals from the body and helps build strong immunity. Free radicals are unstable molecules that can disrupt normal cell function. Vitamin D also helps the immune system, muscles and the nervous system. It also can help to regulate calcium in the body. Vitamin E is a potent antioxidant boosting immune function by removing free radicals. Specific vitamins may be required for particular cancers. Seek out expert help.

Intermittent fasting

Periodic fasting has been practised throughout recorded history. It rests the digestive system allowing it to rebalance and reduce inflammation. Fasting causes cells to move into a type of hibernation and protective mode. Studies have also shown fasting before and after chemo reduces side effects and protects healthy cells while exposing cancerous cells to the treatment. Emerging research indicates intermittent fasting is a powerful approach to reducing cancerous activity. Caution is urged with fasting for advanced cancer patients because of the risks of cachexia.

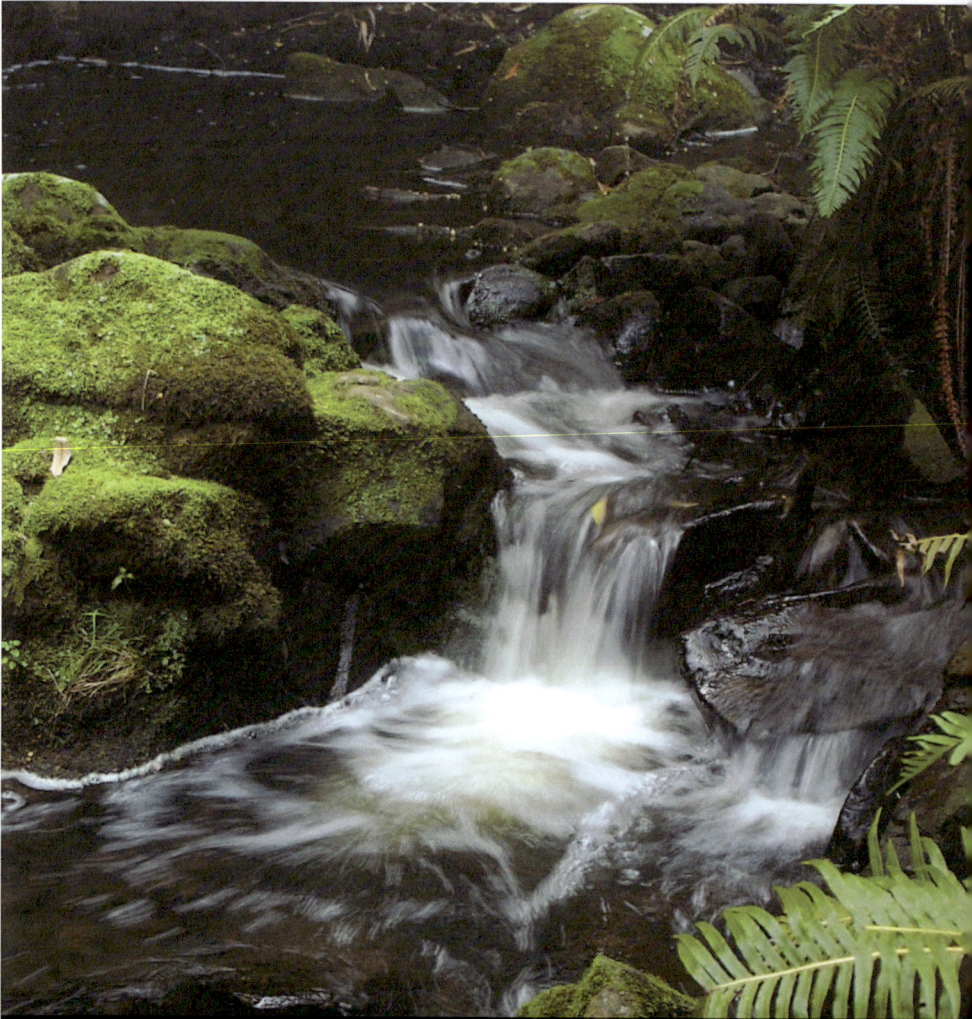

If there is magic on this planet, it is contained in water

Loren Eiseley

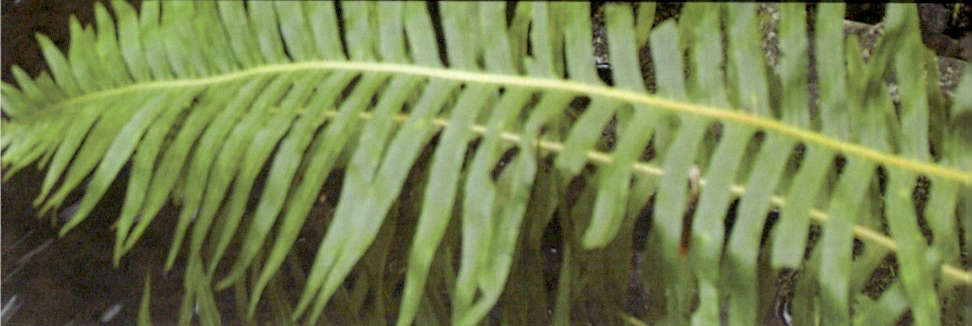

Water

We're often told to drink more water. It's one of the simplest ways of maintaining health but it's easy to forget to do it. The standard recommendation is around eight glasses per day but this depends on many factors. When you exercise you will need more water. Tea and coffee can be included even though they have a slight diuretic effect. Only drink freshly squeezed juices or those from a masticating juicer. Avoid sugary drinks.

The human body is about 60% water and as we know it's essential to every cell's function in our body. It increases energy and relieves fatigue, improves brain function, keeps the digestive system functioning effectively, reduces constipation, helps maintain weight balance, flushes out toxins, helps regulate body temperature, improves skin complexion, cushions joints and helps many other bodily functions. Even mild dehydration creates significant problems in our bodies leading to cognitive issues and increased inflammation.

Ceramic filter

It's best to filter drinking water using a quality ceramic filter. This filters out any potential water-borne contaminants. This may include heavy metals such as arsenic, cadmium, chromium, copper, nickel, lead, aluminium and mercury. It can also remove any bacteria, chlorine, fluoride, glyphosate and other residues.

Much of our food is produced using highly toxic pesticides and herbicides such as Glyphosate (Roundup), antibiotics and hormones. Some of these chemicals find their way into our waterways. Residues may also be on our foods so it's best to wash using filtered water before consuming.

Herbal teas have many health benefits including helping to stay hydrated.

RECIPES *for Success - (organic if possible)*

The Mediterranean Diet

Renowned for its rich flavours and health benefits, the Mediterranean Diet promotes overall well-being through an abundance of fruits, vegetables, whole grains, legumes, nuts, and seeds. Olive oil, a staple, provides heart-healthy monounsaturated fats, reducing cardiovascular risk. Moderate fish and poultry consumption, with limited red meat, ensures balanced protein intake, supporting muscle health and lowering the risk of chronic conditions.

Beyond its physiological advantages, the diet positively influences mental well-being, enhancing cognitive function and lowering the risk of neurodegenerative diseases. The inclusion of omega-3 fatty acids from fish contributes to brain health, potentially reducing cognitive decline. Overall, the Mediterranean Diet's holistic approach nourishes the body and supports a balanced, sustainable lifestyle, making it a well-regarded choice for health promotion.

Plant-based diet

Similarly, a plant-based diet, centered around fruits, vegetables, whole grains, legumes, nuts, and seeds, has demonstrated advantages in reducing the risk of heart disease, diabetes, and cancer. The flexibility of the Flexitarian Diet, which predominantly emphasises plant-based foods but allows occasional consumption of meat and animal products, provides a balanced approach catering to diverse preferences.

DASH and other Diets

Dietary plans such as the DASH (Dietary Approaches to Stop Hypertension) Diet, are specifically designed to manage hypertension (high blood pressure), focus on whole foods, including fruits, vegetables, lean proteins, and whole grains while limiting salt intake. Traditional Japanese or Okinawan diets, rich in vegetables, fish, and soy products, showcase longevity and lower rates of chronic diseases.

Recipes

The recipes on the following pages are based on the above diets and provide a sound starting point for further exploration in healthy eating. In essence, a balanced and varied diet, complemented by regular physical activity, remains fundamental to overall health and well-being.

Bon Appétit!

46

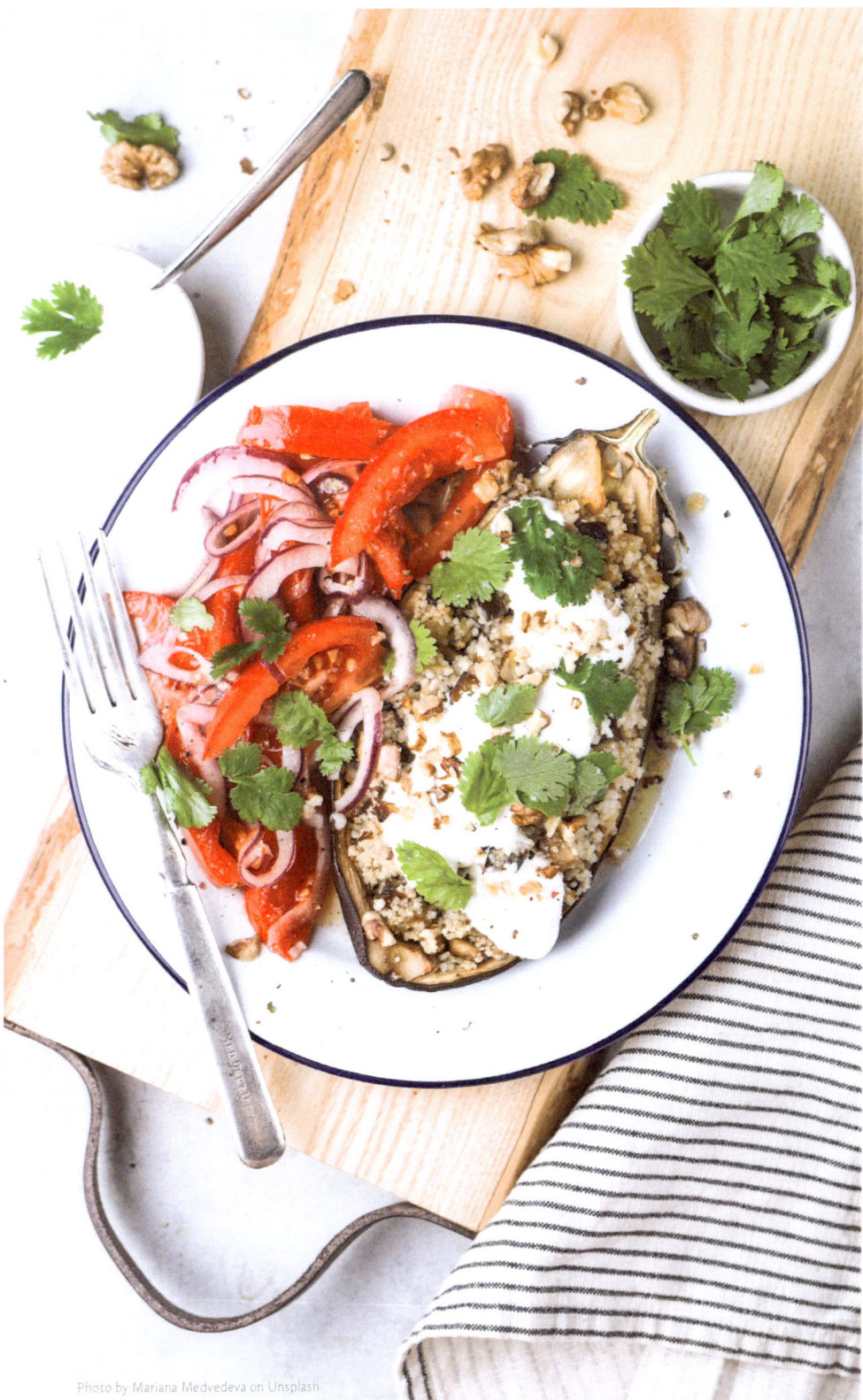

RECIPES *for Success*

Muesli - *Delight*

Start your day with a delicious serving of healthy muesli, yoghurt, fruit, berries and nuts topped with coconut shavings and crushed pistachio nuts.

- Muesli (your own style as long as it's low in sugar and high in unprocessed ingredients). A healthy alternative is quinoa or brown rice flakes

- Sprinkle hemp seed

- Add sliced fruit (banana, pear, apple etc.). Fresh, seasonal is best. Choose the best quality natural fruits that are available (or in containers, choose ones with no preservatives and only natural sugars).

- Add berries (strawberries, blueberries, cranberries, currants etc.)

- A dollop of organic coconut yoghurt

- Sprinkle sunflower and pumpkin seeds, coconut flakes and crushed nuts (including pistachio)

- A drizzle of honey (if sweetness required)

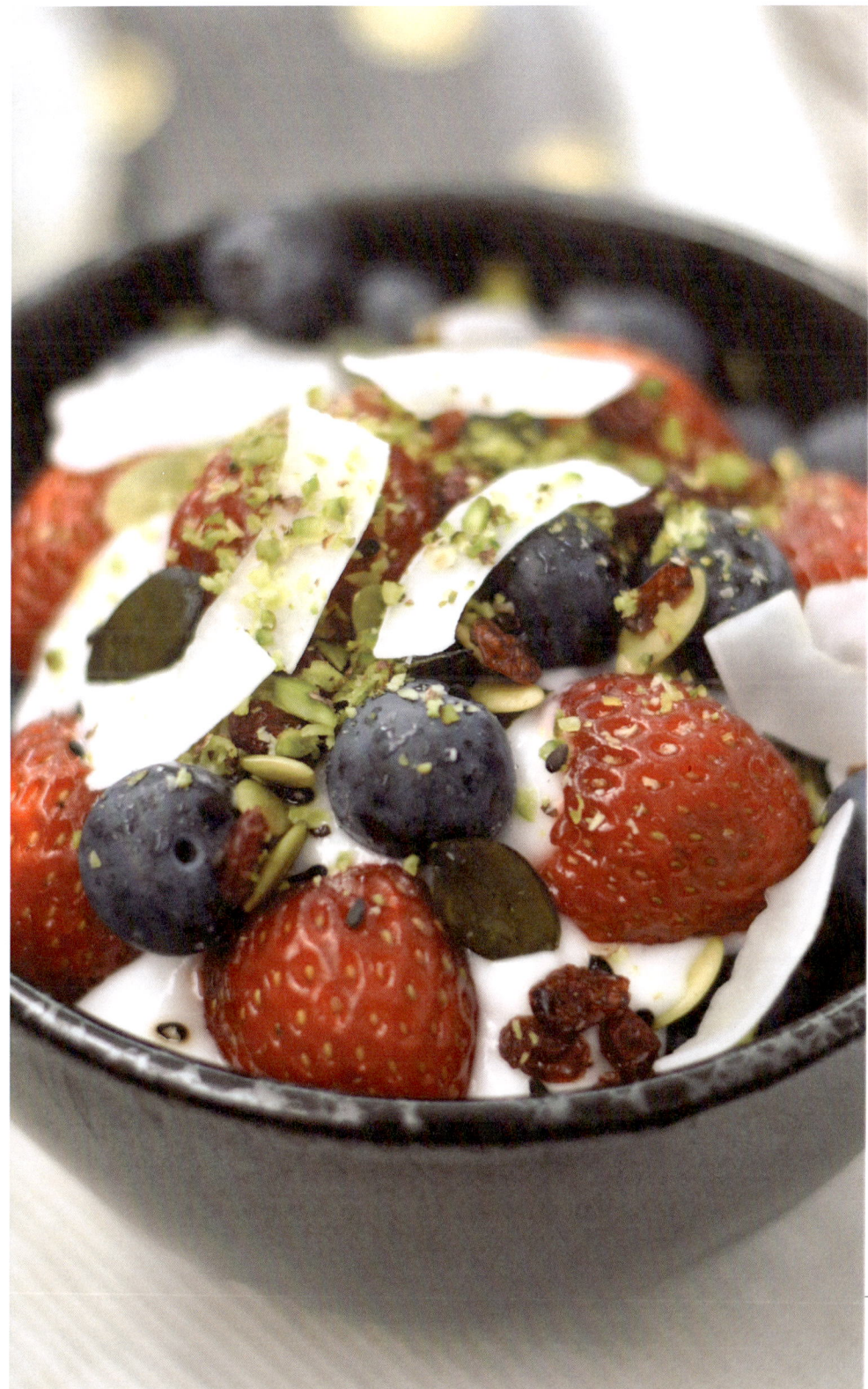

Lunchtime - *Zing*

Choose a delicious, wholesome, fresh, spelt buckwheat and polenta crusty bread slice and add avocado and a spoonful of garlic paste. Add spinach leaves, tomato, onion, beetroot and beanshoots (homegrown) from the garden. Sprinkle with dukkah and turmeric and top with a tasty lettuce leaf. *Yum!*

- Fresh spelt buckwheat and polenta crusty bread slice (or, whatever wholesome bread you can find!)

- Avocado (spread) with a touch of garlic paste

- Spinach leaves, tomato, onion and beetroot

- Beanshoots (easy to grow your own - packed with incredible nutrition)

- Sprinkle with dukkah and turmeric

- Top with some lettuce leaves from the garden

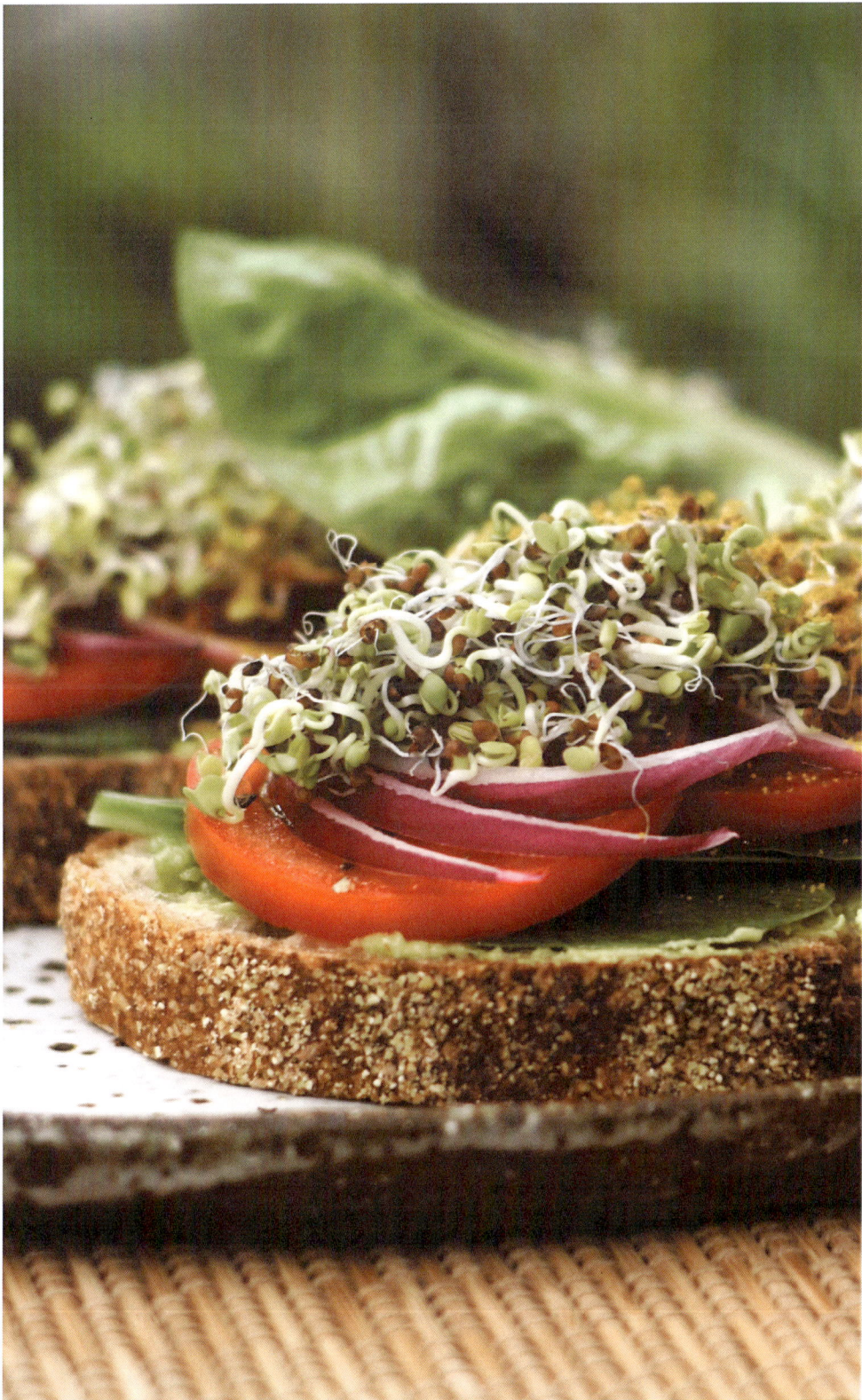

Poached Egg, Sliced Chips and Salad

A quick and easy pick-me-up snack,
balancing taste, texture and nutrition.

- 1 egg (poached)
- 1 tbsp (20ml) white-wine vinegar
- 1 desiree potato, peeled and thinly sliced, using a mandoline
- 2-3 thin slices of red capsicum
- Cherry tomatoes
- Baby coz lettuce leaves
- Chilly flakes

Dressing

- 1 tbsp extra-virgin olive oil
- 1 tsp (5ml) lemon juice
- 1 small garlic clove, crushed

Preheat the oven to 180°C. Stack the potato slices and place onto baking paper and drizzle with oil. Bake for 30-35 minutes, or until golden.

Whisk all dressing ingredients together.

Fill a saucepan with water and bring to boil. Simmer gently. Add the vinegar. Swirl into a whirlpool and gently add the egg into the middle. Cook for 3 minutes then remove with a slotted spoon. Dry with a clean white tea towel.

Place lettuce leaves, capsicum slices and potato stack onto a plate. Gently place the egg onto the potato stack. Pour the dressing onto the egg and chips. Sprinkle chilly flakes.

Serves 1

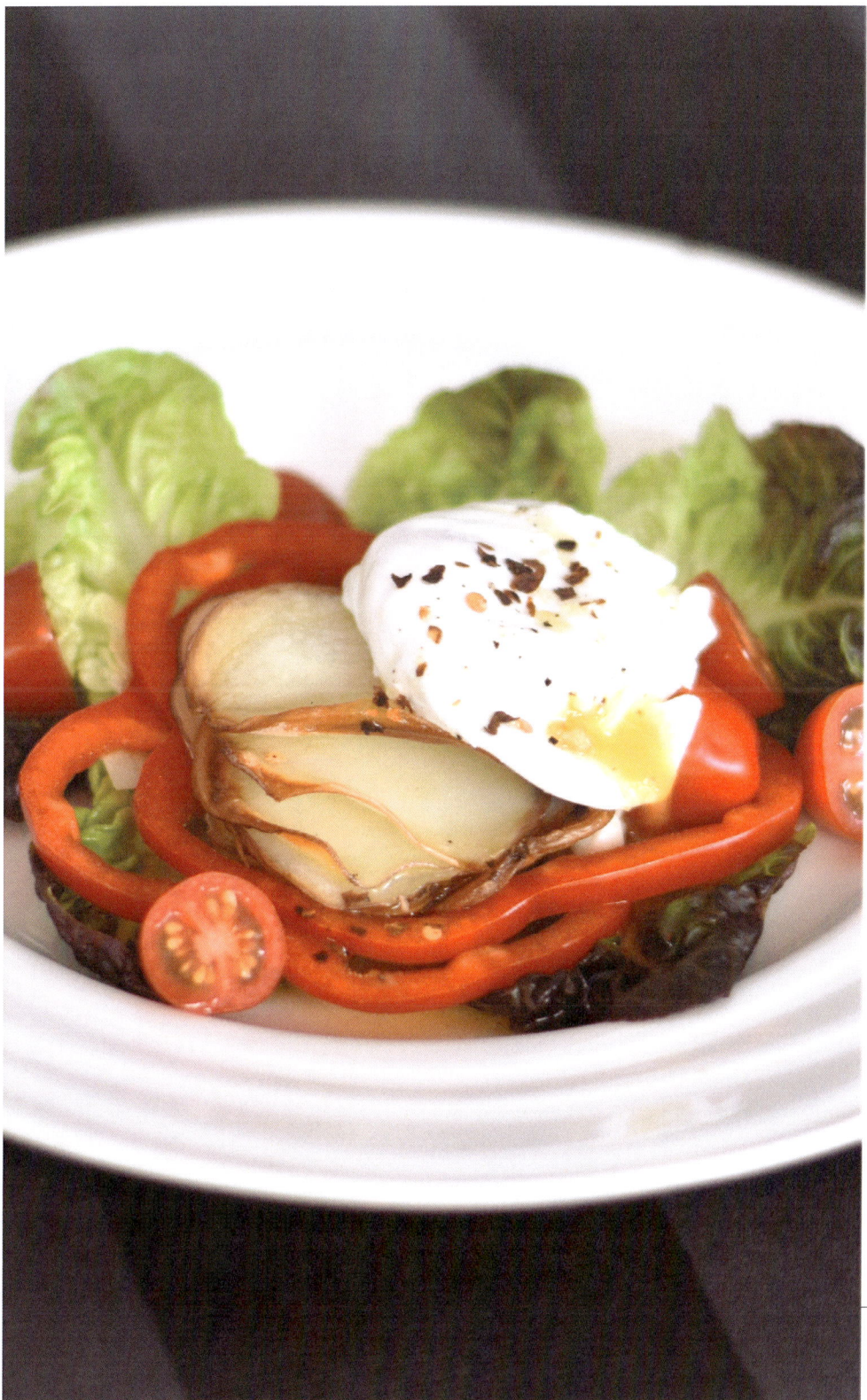

Berry Nice Juice

Fresh, colourful and unprocessed fruits and vegetables naturally contain phytochemicals which provide us with rich antioxidants that boost our immune function. This berry juice has a delightful hit of flavour, rich in antioxidants, particularly vitamins A and C.

Your immune system will love you!

- 1 cup strawberries (100g)
- ½ cup raspberries (50g)
- ½ cup cranberries (50g)
- ½ pear (150g)

Use a quality slow juicer. Wash all ingredients. Cut pear into chunks. Add all ingredients into juicer. Keep the pulp in the refrigerator and add to muesli the next morning.

Serves 1

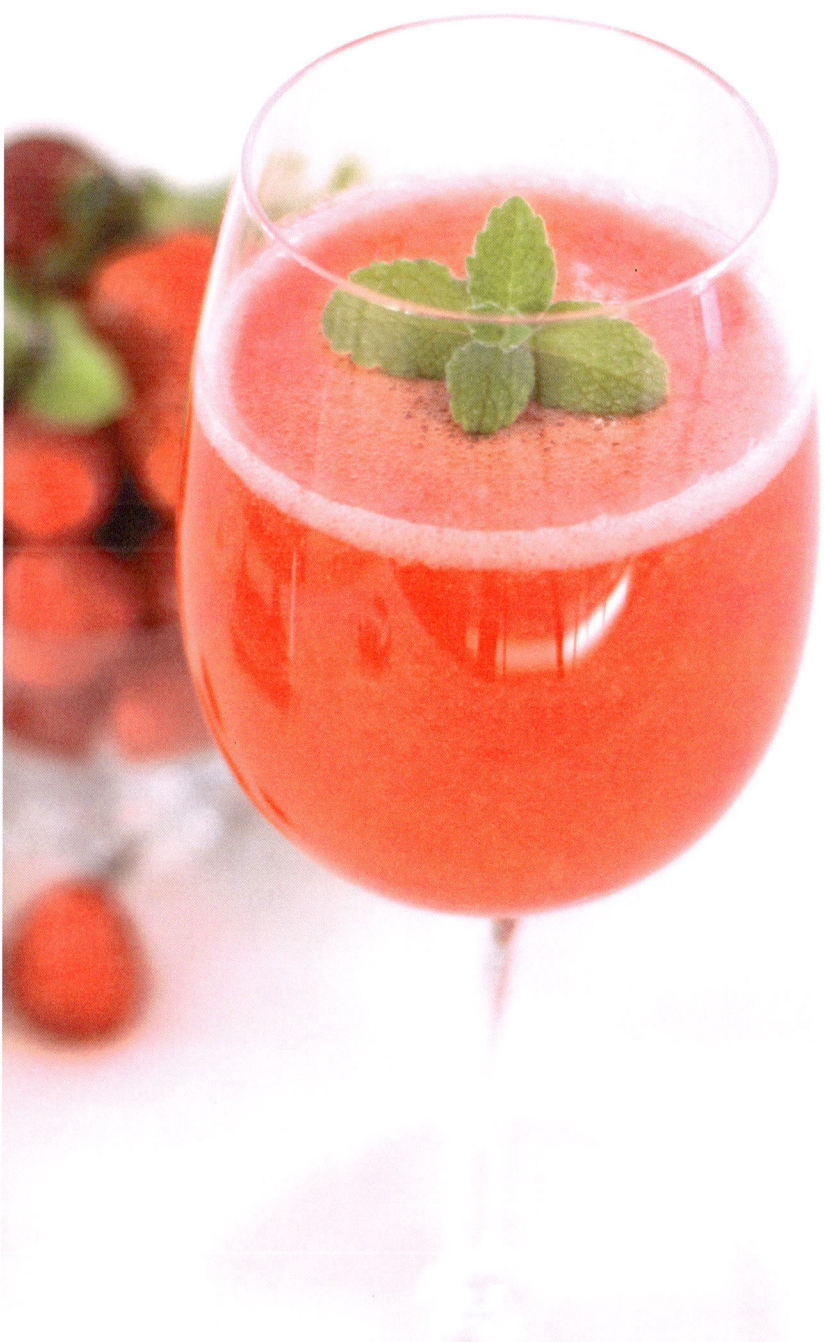

Clean Green Juice

This detoxifying and soothing juice is packed with nutrition. The apples add sweetness to the balance.

- 2 apples (180g x 2)
- A handful of spinach (50g)
- 1 kale leaf (20g)
- 1 small ginger piece (20g)
- ½ cucumber (90g)
- ½ green capsicum (60g)
- ¼ lemon (30g)

Soak the spinach and kale for 10-15 minutes in cold water before juicing. This will help release the optimal nutrients.

Use a quality slow juicer. Wash all ingredients. Remove the stem and seeds from the capsicum. Add all ingredients slowly into the juicer.

Serves 1

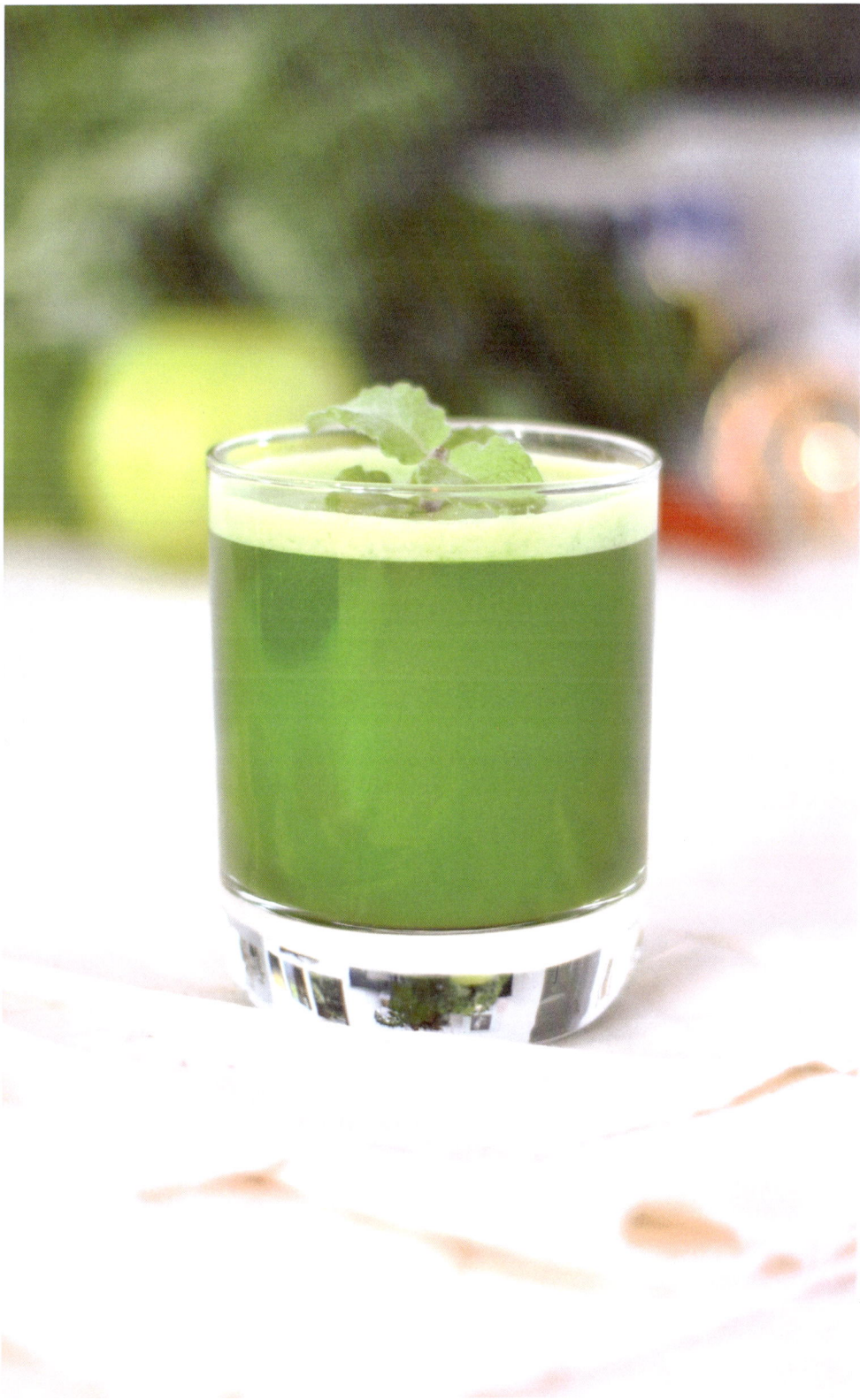

Crazy Cool Carrot Juice

The rich colour indicates the high levels of the antioxidant, beta-carotene. It's also packed with many other vitamins and minerals which enhances your immune system.

- 4 carrots (160g x 4)

Soak the carrots for 30 minutes in cold water before juicing. This will help release the optimal nutrients.

Use a quality slow juicer. Wash all ingredients. Remove the carrot tops and cut into sections to fit the juicer. Slowly add all ingredients into the juicer.

Serves 1

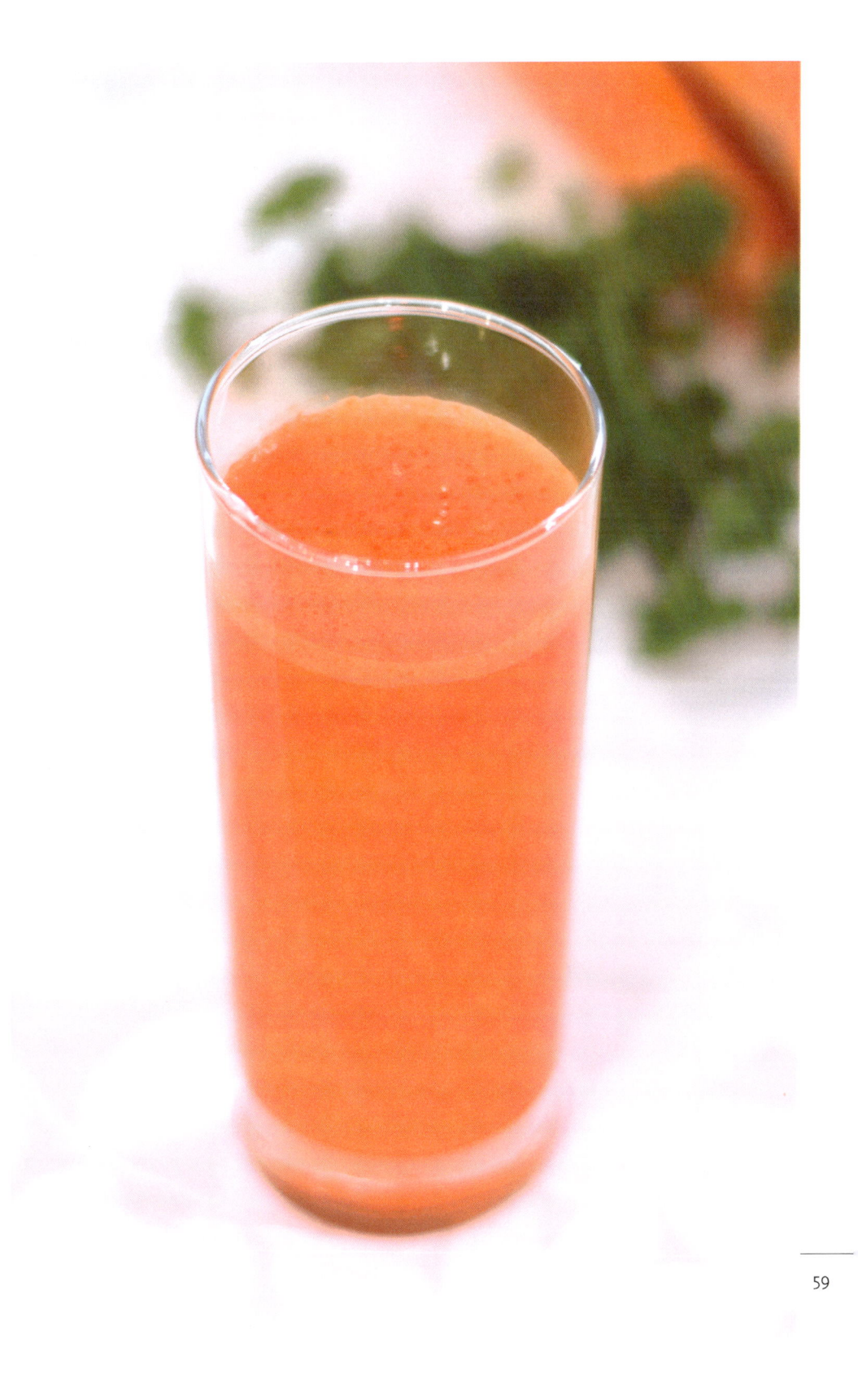

Green Barley Salad and Goat's Cheese

Seasonal, fresh produce (ideally from your own garden) can be combined into a delicious green salad with pearl barley and goat's cheese. You can also add a cup of broad beans or other greens to the mix, as desired.

- 3 cups (750ml) water
- 1 cup (250g) pearl barley
- 1 cup (120g) peas
- 150g green beans, trimmed, halved lengthways
- 1 Lebanese cucumber (130g) halved lengthways, sliced thinly
- 1 baby coz lettuce, trimmed, torn
- 2 spring onions, sliced thinly
- 1 cup fresh mint leaves
- 2 tbsp extra virgin olive oil
- 1 tbsp lemon juice
- 150g goat's cheese

Place the barley and water into a medium saucepan, bring to the boil and reduce to a low heat. Simmer covered for 35 minutes or until tender. Drain, rinse under cold water until cool.

Meanwhile, cook peas and beans in a large saucepan for 2 minutes or until tender; drain and run under cold water until cool. Blanching peas and beans briefly, helps retain their bright colour. If adding broad beans, remove the outer shell, keep grey skin intact during blanching then remove once cool.

Transfer barley, peas and beans into a large bowl. Add cucumber, lettuce, spring onion and mint. Combine oil and juice and drizzle over the top. Gently toss to combine. Crumble goat's cheese on top and add pepper to taste.

Serves 6

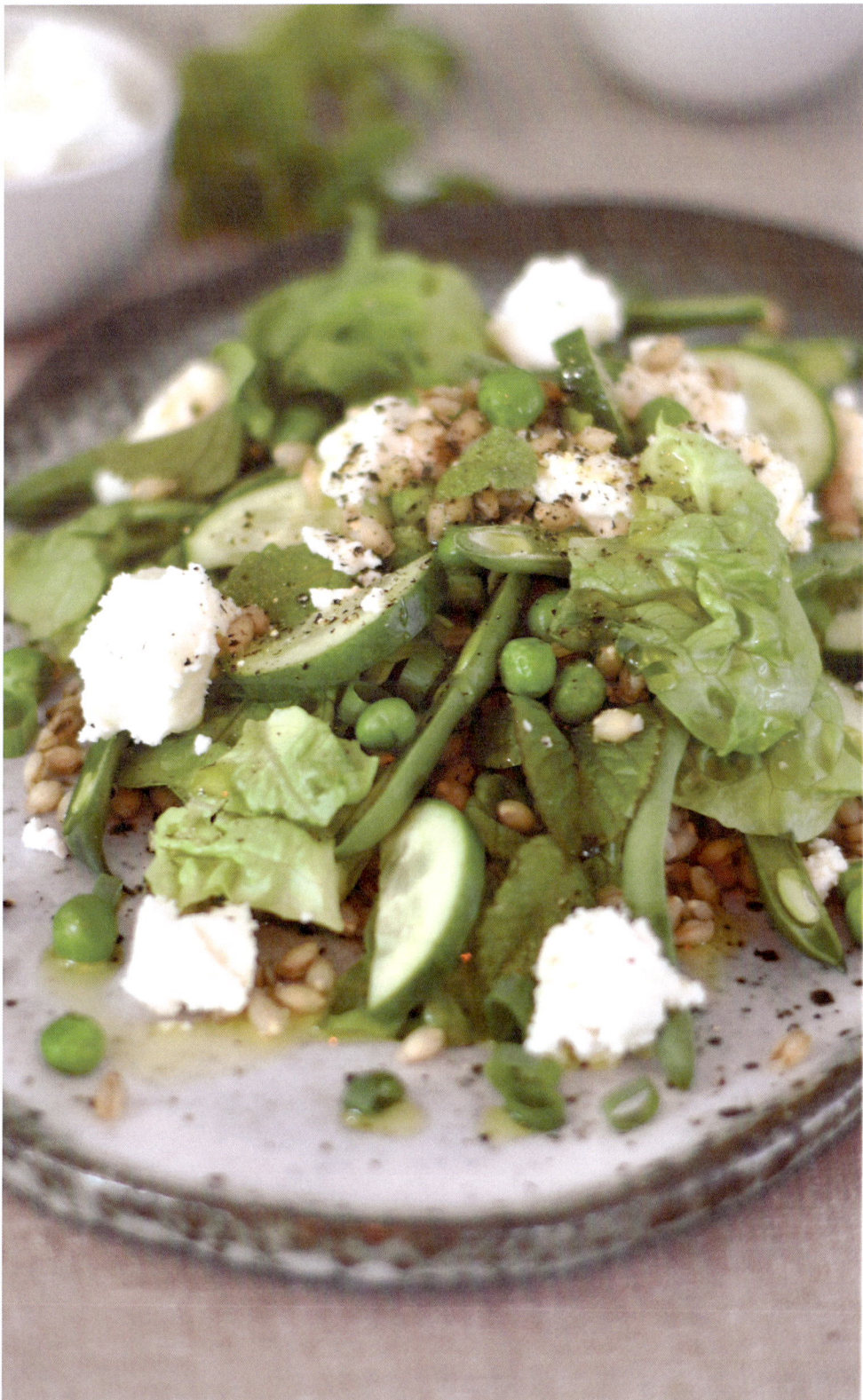

Blood Orange Pistachio Quinoa

Quinoa is a super healing food containing multiple essential amino acids. It's a great base for so many other flavours and textures. The blood orange, cranberries and pistachio adds a great depth of flavour and goodness.

- 1½ cups quinoa
- 1 blood orange, segmented, all pith carefully sliced off
- ½ cup pistachios (shelled)
- 2½ cups water
- 1 tsp cumin
- ½ cup fresh coriander, finely shredded
- ⅛ tsp pepper
- ½ cup mint leaves, chopped
- 2 spring onions, finely chopped
- Zest of 1 orange
- ⅛ cup orange juice
- 1½ tbsp olive oil
- 1½ tbsp lemon juice
- ½ cup cranberries, each chopped roughly in half

Place the quinoa in a fine mesh container and rinse well to remove the natural bitter resin. Place in a pot, bring to the boil then simmer for 15 minutes. Remove from heat and fluff with a fork. Spread on a baking dish and continue to fluff occasionally with a fork until cool.

Meanwhile, lightly roast the pistachios by spreading them on a baking dish, heat the oven to 150°C and bake for 7-10 mins until slightly browned.

Transfer quinoa into a large bowl and add cumin, coriander, mint, spring onions, orange juice, olive oil, lemon juice, toasted pistachios and cranberries. Mix well.

Spoon onto a serving plate. Evenly distribute the blood orange segments and gently mix them in. Sprinkle the orange zest and mint leaves and add pepper to taste.

Serves 6

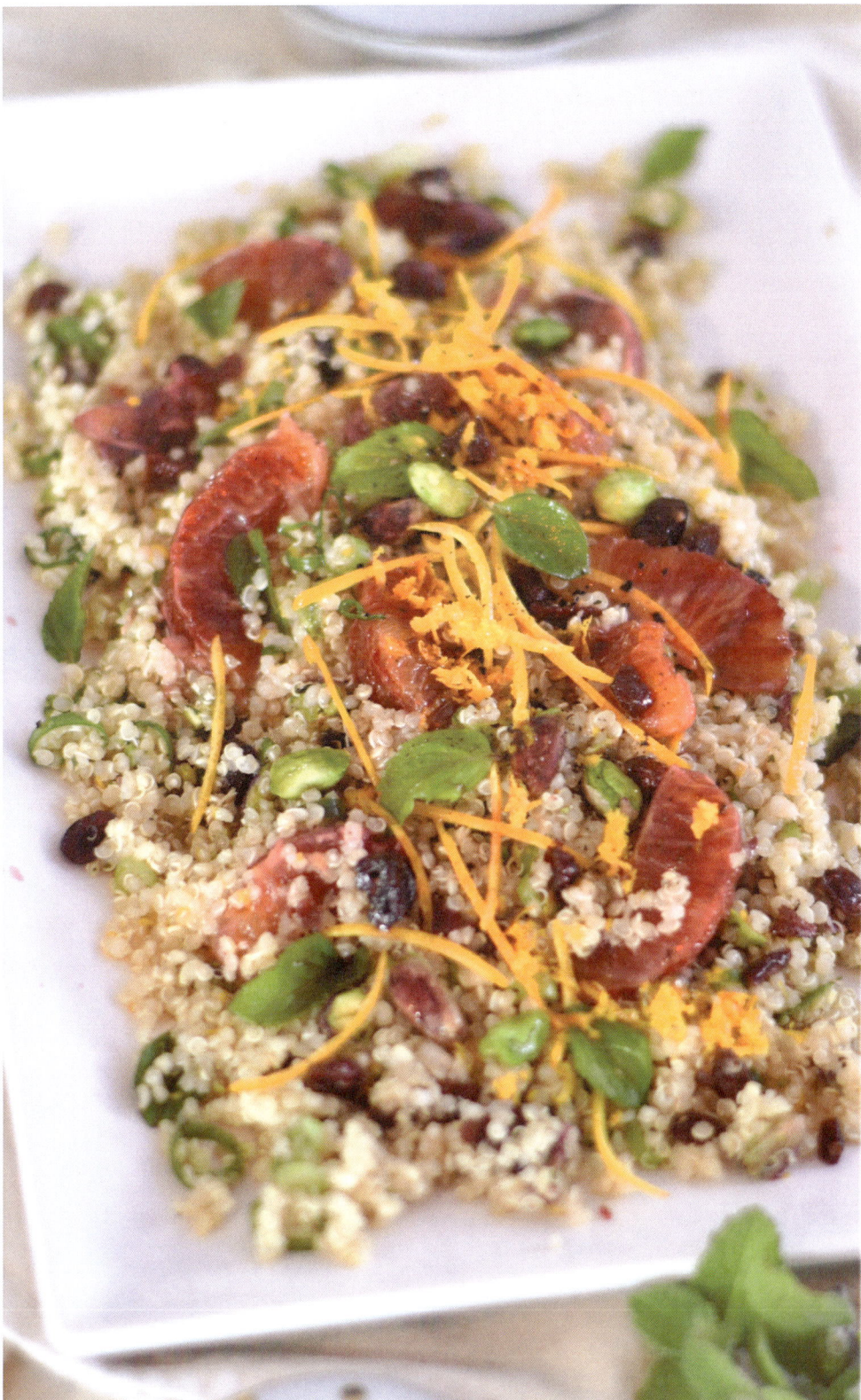

Healing Broth

Perfect for providing valuable minerals in an easy to drink broth. Ideal after treatments to enhance the healing process. It can be used as a drink on it's own or as a starting point for a variety of soups. The magnesium, potassium and sodium rejuvenates the body.

- 2 unpeeled red potatoes, quartered
- 1 unpeeled onion, cut into chunks
- 3 unpeeled carrots, cut into thirds
- 1 unpeeled sweet potato, quartered
- 1 leek, cut into thirds
- ½ bunch of celery, cut into thirds
- 3 unpeeled cloves garlic, halved
- ¼ bunch fresh parsley
- 1 strip of kombu (seaweed)
- 4 litres of filtered water

Thoroughly rinse all of the vegetables and kombu and place into a large saucepan of filtered water. Bring to boil. Remove the lid and simmer for at least 2 hours (the longer it simmers, the richer the flavours!). Add more water if needed to keep all vegetables constantly immersed.

Strain the broth using a coarse sieve and serve. Once cooled, it can also be frozen in smaller containers.

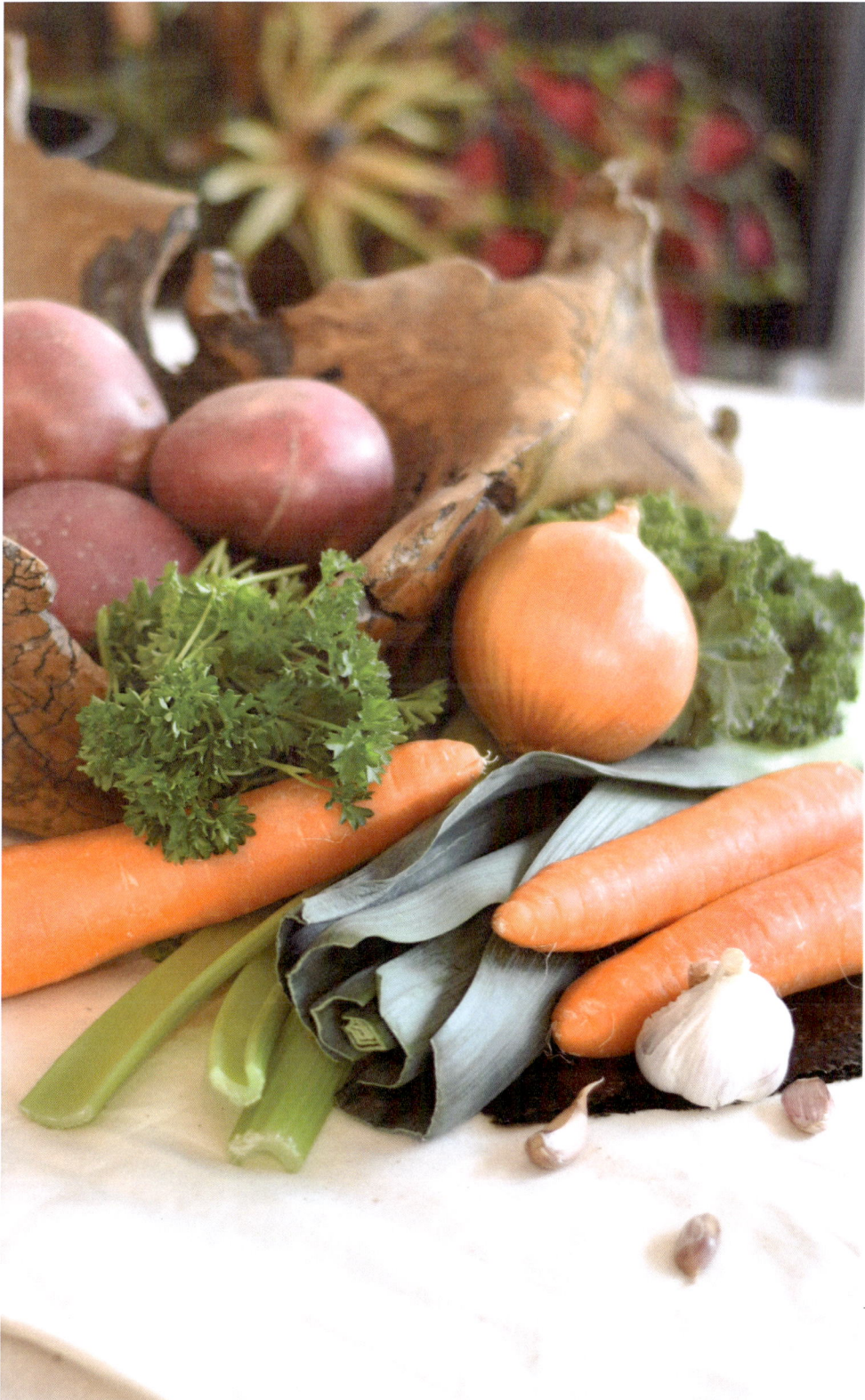

Pumpkin and Feta, Oven-baked Risotto

Share this warming, healthy, delicious and easy to prepare, oven-baked dish.

- 3 tsp extra virgin olive oil
- 1 leek finely chopped
- 2 garlic cloves, crushed
- 500g pumpkin, peeled, diced into 1cm pieces
- Zest of 1 lemon
- 1 tbsp chopped thyme leaves
- 5 tbsp (100ml) dry white wine
- 900ml vegetable stock
- 250g brown rice
- ½ cup peas
- 100g feta, crumbled
- Baby rocket leaves, to serve

Preheat oven to 200°C.

Add the olive oil to a large flameproof dish over medium-high heat. Cook the leek for 2-3 minutes until soft. Add the garlic, and cook for a further minute. Remove from heat.

Add stock, rice, wine and half the lemon zest. Cover with tight-fitting tinfoil and bake on a middle shelf in the oven, stirring every 15 minutes for 35 minutes or until rice is tender and liquid is absorbed.

Meanwhile, place pumpkin on a baking tray. Drizzle with oil and season with pepper. Bake on top shelf of the oven for 30 minutes.

Once all is cooked, add pumpkin and peas to the risotto and gently stir to combine. To serve, divide the risotto among serving bowls. Crumble feta on top and sprinkle with the remaining lemon zest and add baby rocket leaves to garnish. For extra zing and colour, garnish with finely cut chilli.

Serves 6

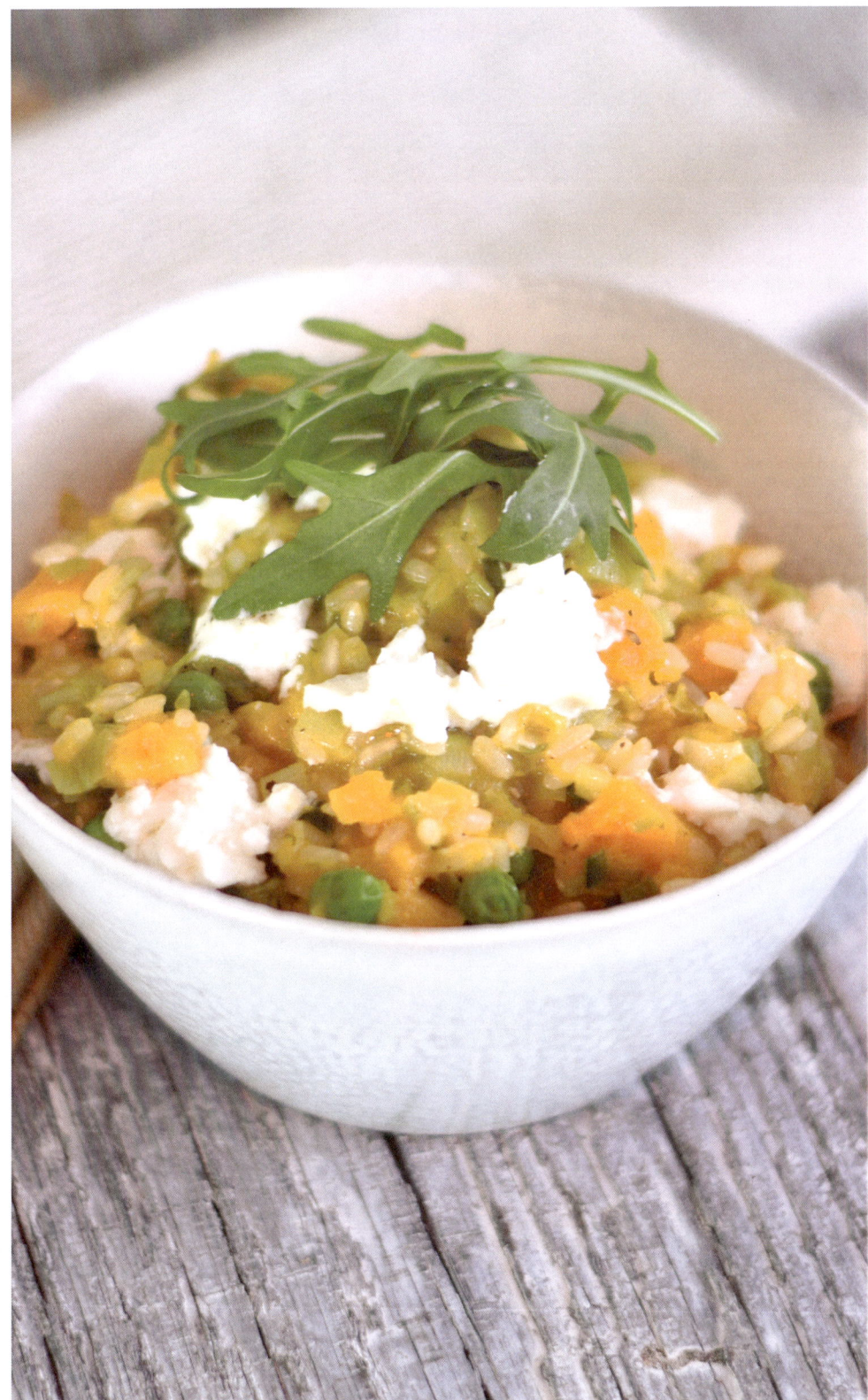

Asparagus, Potato and Goat's Cheese Frittata

High in folate, Vitamin K, minerals and antioxidants, the healthy asparagus features in both the aesthetics and rich nutrient value in this dish.

- 800g starchy potatoes, peeled and cut into wedges
- 2 tbsp olive oil
- 10-12 spears asparagus, halved using angles slices
- 6 eggs
- 1 cup (250ml) cooking cream
- ⅓ cup (25g) grated parmesan
- 100g goat's cheese, crumbled

Preheat the oven to 210°C. Place the potatoes and oil into a 1.5 litre (6 cup) ceramic baking dish and toss to coat. Bake for 45 minutes or until golden. Top with the asparagus. Place the eggs, cream, parmesan into a bowl and whisk to combine. Pour over the potatoes and asparagus and crumble the goat's cheese on top.

Bake for 20-30 minutes until the top is golden. Cover with tinfoil to prevent the top from overcooking. Continue to cook for another 30-35 minutes until filling is thoroughly cooked.

Serves 4

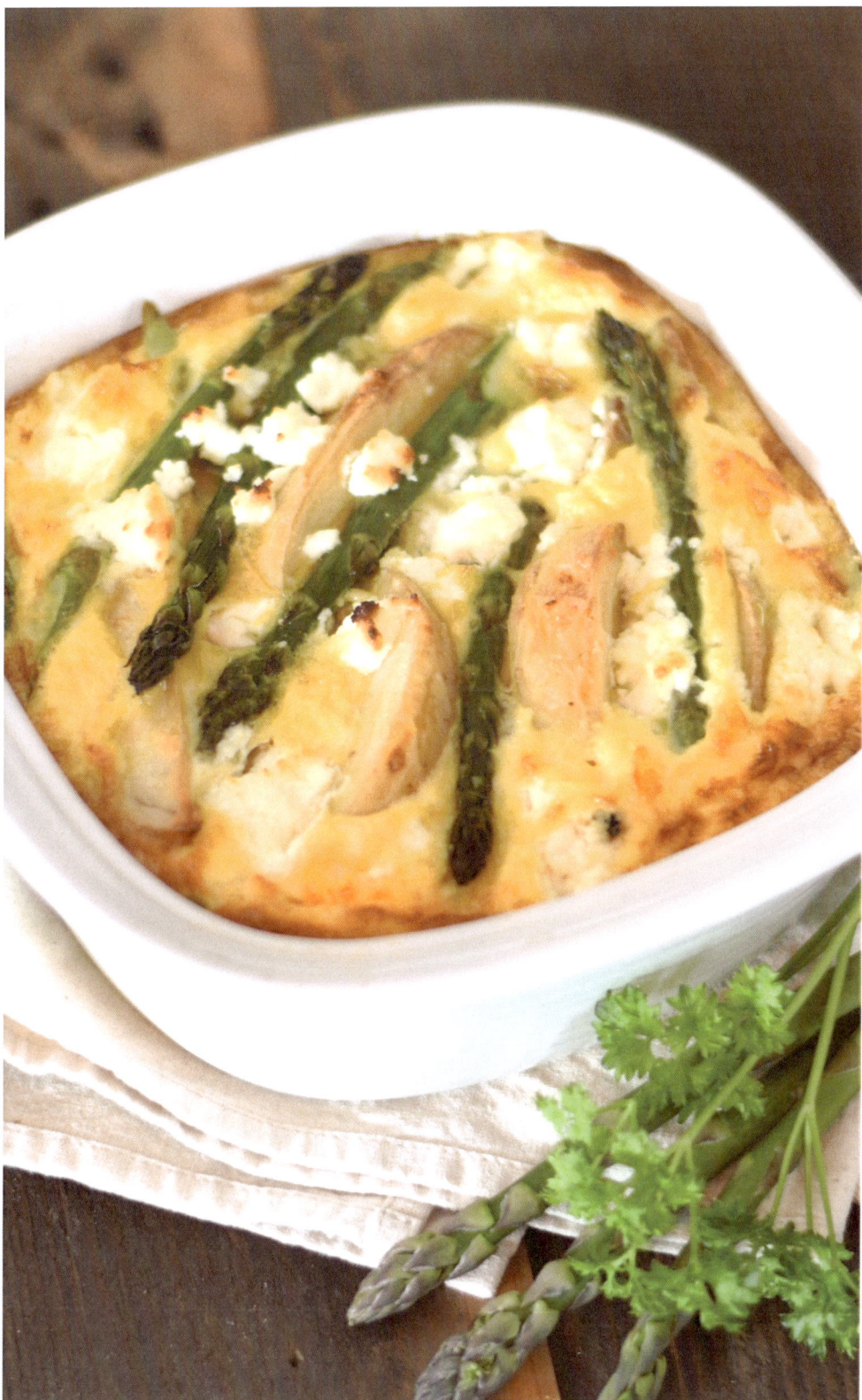

Spinach (or Silverbeet/Kale) and Feta Pie

Indulge in this Spinach and Feta Pie for a taste of wholesome goodness! Packed with nutrient-rich spinach (or silverbeet/kale) and creamy feta, this savoury delight promises a delectable fusion of flavour and health benefits in every bite.

- 1kg spinach or a combination of spinach/silverbeet/kale
- Olive oil
- 6 spring onions, finely chopped
- 6 eggs
- 125g feta cheese, crumbled
- 90g grated cheddar cheese
- 16 sheets filo pastry
- 1 tbsp poppy seeds

Preheat the oven to 210°C. Grease a 25 x 30cm baking dish. Wash the spinach and shred finely. Place in a large saucepan and cover. Cook on low heat until just wilted. Allow to cool, squeeze out excess water and dry with clean tea towel.

Gently cook the spring onion in a fry pan until soft. Put the onion into a mixing bowl. Add 5 eggs (leave 1 for later!) and lightly beat. Add the spinach and feta and mix thoroughly.

Place one layer of pastry into the baking dish and brush with oil. Add the next 6 layers on top brushing each with oil in the same way.

Add the spinach mix on top of the pastry and fold the edges in. Add the remaining pastry sheets brushing each with oil. Tuck down the sides.

Lightly beat the last egg and brush all over the top. Sprinkle the poppy seeds on top.

Bake for 15-20 minutes until the pastry is golden. Cover with tinfoil. Continue to cook for another 30-35 minutes until filling is thoroughly cooked.

Serves 6-8 (freezes well)

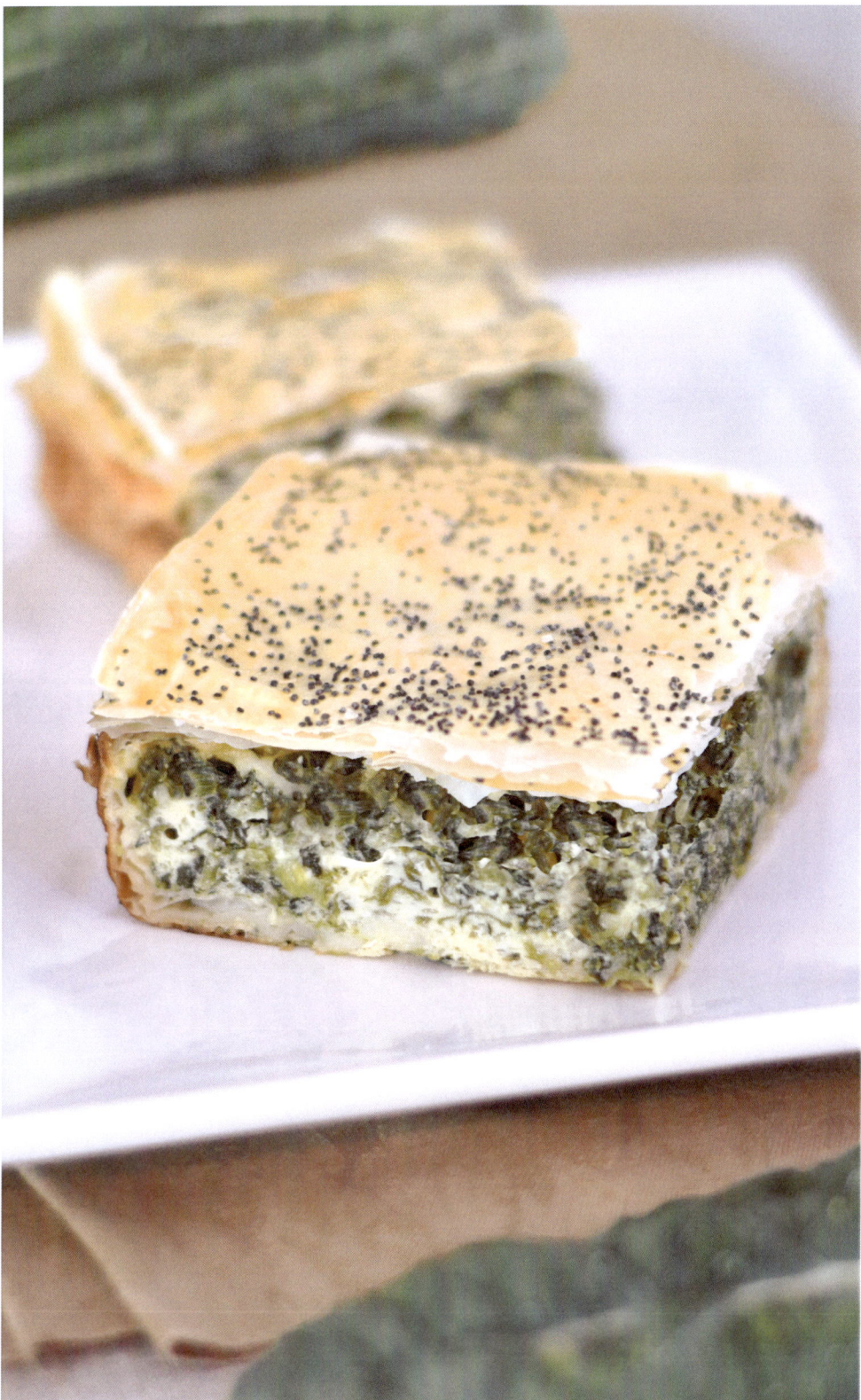

Pan-fried Fish with Black-bean Dressing

Fish is rich in calcium and phosphorus and a great source of minerals, such as iron, zinc, iodine, magnesium and potassium. It's best eaten at least twice a week.

- 8 x 150g fish fillets
- 2 tbsp buckwheat flour, seasoned with pepper
- 2 tbsp (40ml) extra virgin olive oil
- Brown rice to serve

Black-bean dressing
- 2 tsp fish sauce and sesame oil
- 1 tsp light soy sauce
- 4 tbsp (80ml) olive oil
- Zest and juice of 3 limes
- ¼ cup (3 tbsp) black beans (rinsed)
- 1 long red chilli, seeds removed, thinly sliced
- 1 red onion, thinly sliced
- 2 tbsp chopped coriander, plus extra to serve

Cook the brown rice using preferred method.

Meanwhile, combine all the dressing ingredients (keep some zest for garnishing) and set aside.

Preheat the oven and a baking dish on low heat.

Lightly dust the fish in flour.

Heat the oil in a pan over a medium-low heat and cook the fish for 2 minutes each side, or until golden. Each fillet can then be placed onto the baking dish in the oven on low heat until all fillets are complete.

Serve the rice on each plate and top each with 2 fish fillets.
Pour on the dressing and garnish with extra coriander.

Serves 4

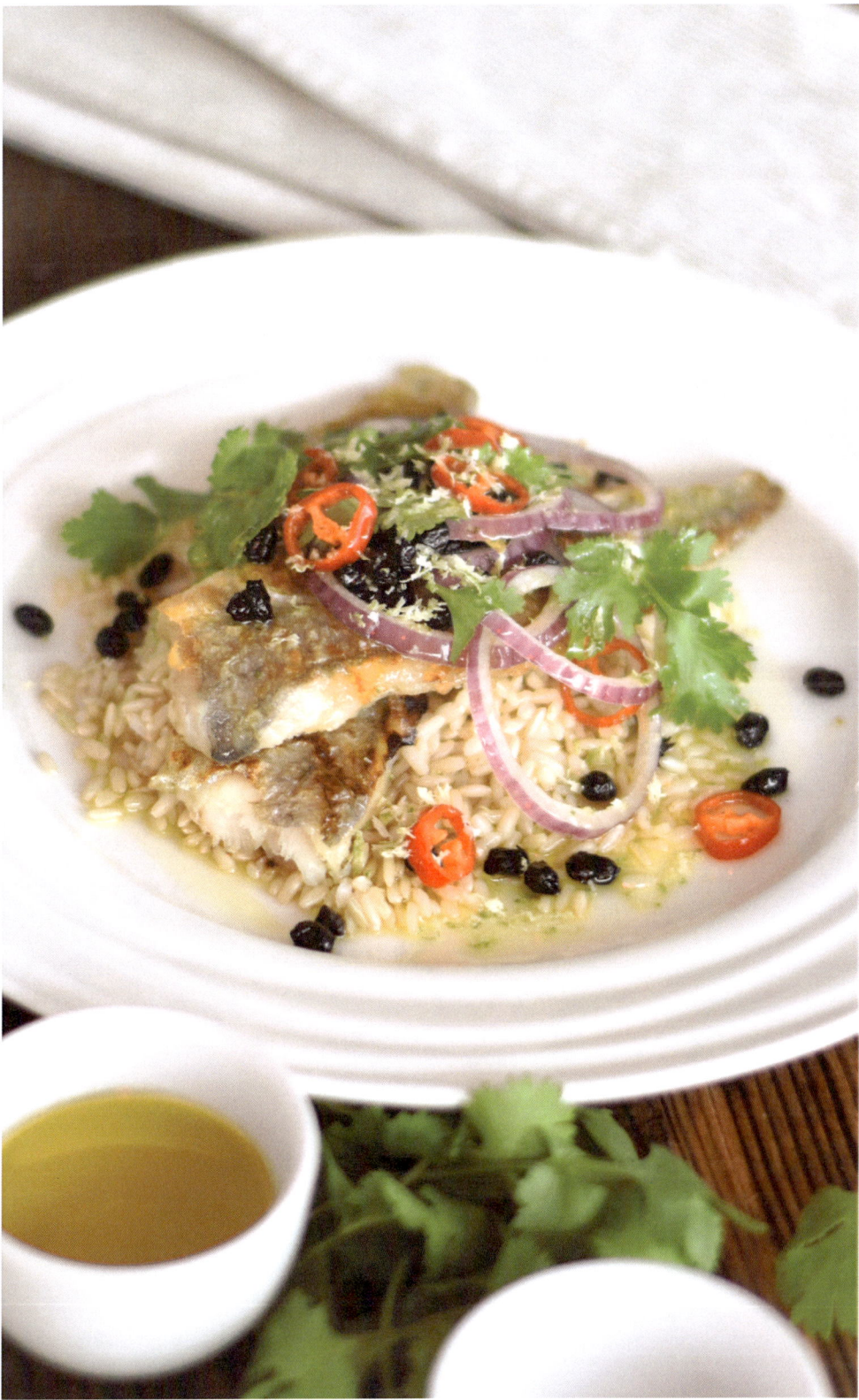

Tuscan Kale Fritters and Beetroot

These delicious and super healthy fritters are rich in fibre, protein, antioxidants, vitamins A, C and K, and folate.

- 3 Tuscan Kale leaves (30g) trimmed and finely shredded
- 3 large zucchinis (450g) coarsely grated
- 2 tbsp chopped mint leaves
- Mint leaves to serve
- 2 cloves of garlic, crushed
- 2 eggs lightly beaten
- ¼ cup (40g) buckwheat flour
- ⅓ cup (80ml) extra virgin olive oil
- 1 tbsp apple cider vinegar
- ½ teaspoon honey
- 100g feta, crumbled
- 2 tbsp sunflower seeds, lightly toasted
- 3 small beets, peeled and thinly sliced (ideally use a mandoline)
- 2 tbsp apple cider vinegar

Place zucchini in a colander over the sink. Using your hand squeeze excess juice from the zucchini.

In a medium bowl combine the zucchini, kale, mint, flour, garlic and egg.

Meanwhile combine beetroot and vinegar in a bowl, stand for 5 minutes then drain into a small bowl to make the dressing. Add the remaining oil, vinegar and honey to the beetroot juice dressing.

Using a non-stick pan over medium heat, add half the oil. Scoop ¼ cups of the mixture into the pan, flattening slightly each time. Cook for 5 minutes each side or until lightly golden. Drain each on paper towel until all are cooked.

Plate up the fritters, top with beetroot slices, crumbled feta and drizzle the dressing. Sprinkle sunflower seeds and mint.

Serves 4

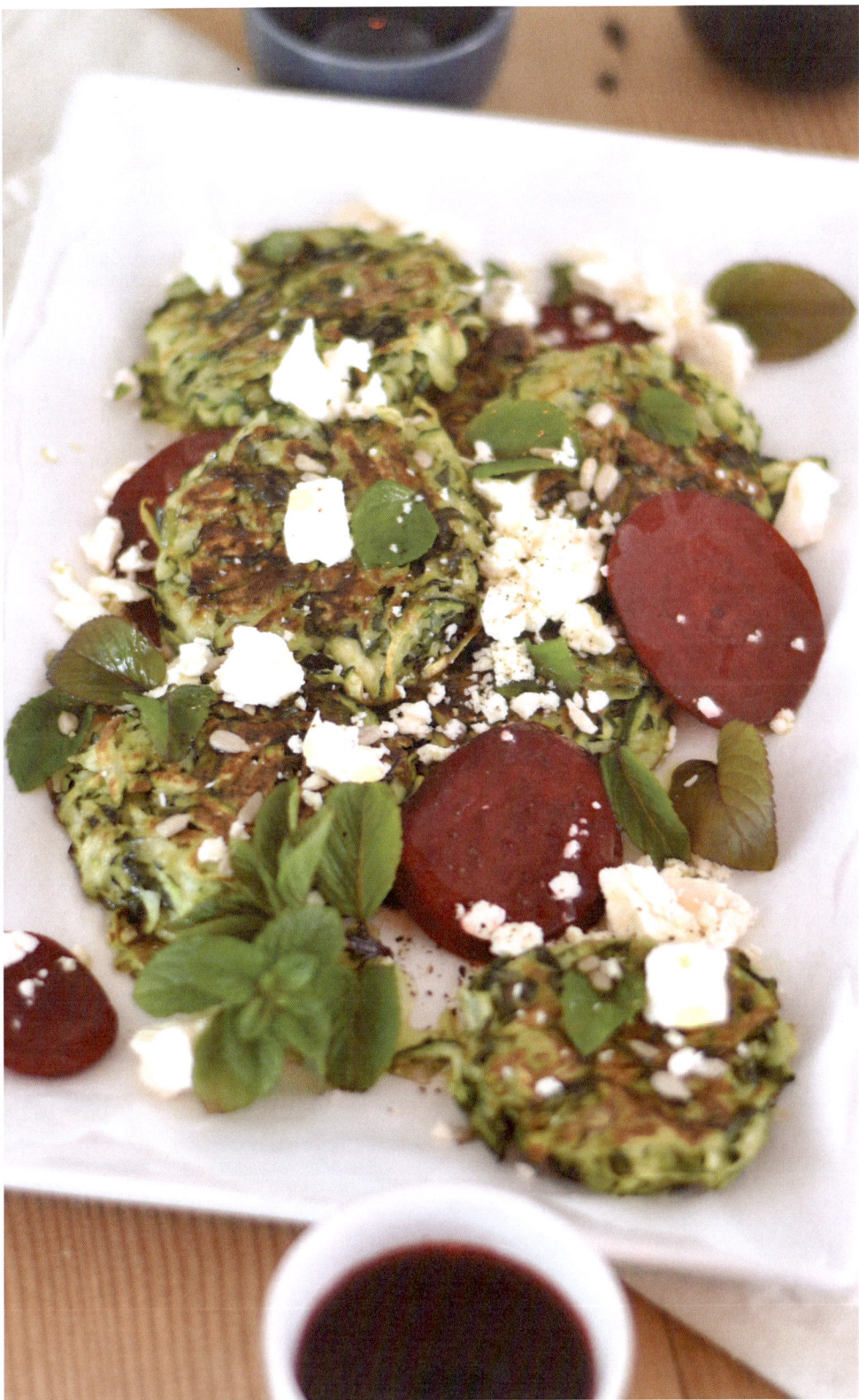

Chilli Chicken Skewers, Avocado Salad and Sweet Potato Noodles

Avocados are a nutritional powerhouse! Packed with essential nutrients like heart-healthy fats and fibre, these creamy delights also boast a wealth of anti-inflammatory and antioxidant compounds. This is a delicious recipe to delight all the family.

- Around 800g chicken breast fillets, cut into pieces
- 100g sweet potato noodles (also called glass noodles, they become translucent once cooked) or use brown rice noodles
- ¼ cup (90g) Asian chilli jam
- 2 Lebanese cucumbers, finely shredded
- 2 zucchini's, finely shredded
- 2 avocados, chopped into small pieces
- 1 cup coriander leaves, plus extra to serve
- 1 small red chilli, thinly sliced, seeds removed

Dressing
- 2 tbsp lime juice
- 1 tbsp fish sauce

Preheat the grill pan or barbeque over high heat. Place the chicken and oil into a large bowl and toss to combine. Thread the chicken onto 8 metal skewers and cook for 5-6 minutes each side or until thoroughly cooked. Brush each skewer with the chilli jam and cook for a further minute on each side. Set aside.

While the chicken is cooking, place the noodles in a large bowl, cover with boiling water and set aside for 2 minutes to soften. Drain, run under cold water and drain again. Add the zucchini, cucumber, coriander and avocado.

For the dressing, combine the lime juice and fish sauce in a small jug and then pour over the noodles and salad.

Plate up the skewers, noodles and salad. Garnish with the sliced chilli and coriander. Crushed nuts can also be sprinkled on top (*be mindful of allergies*).

Serves 4

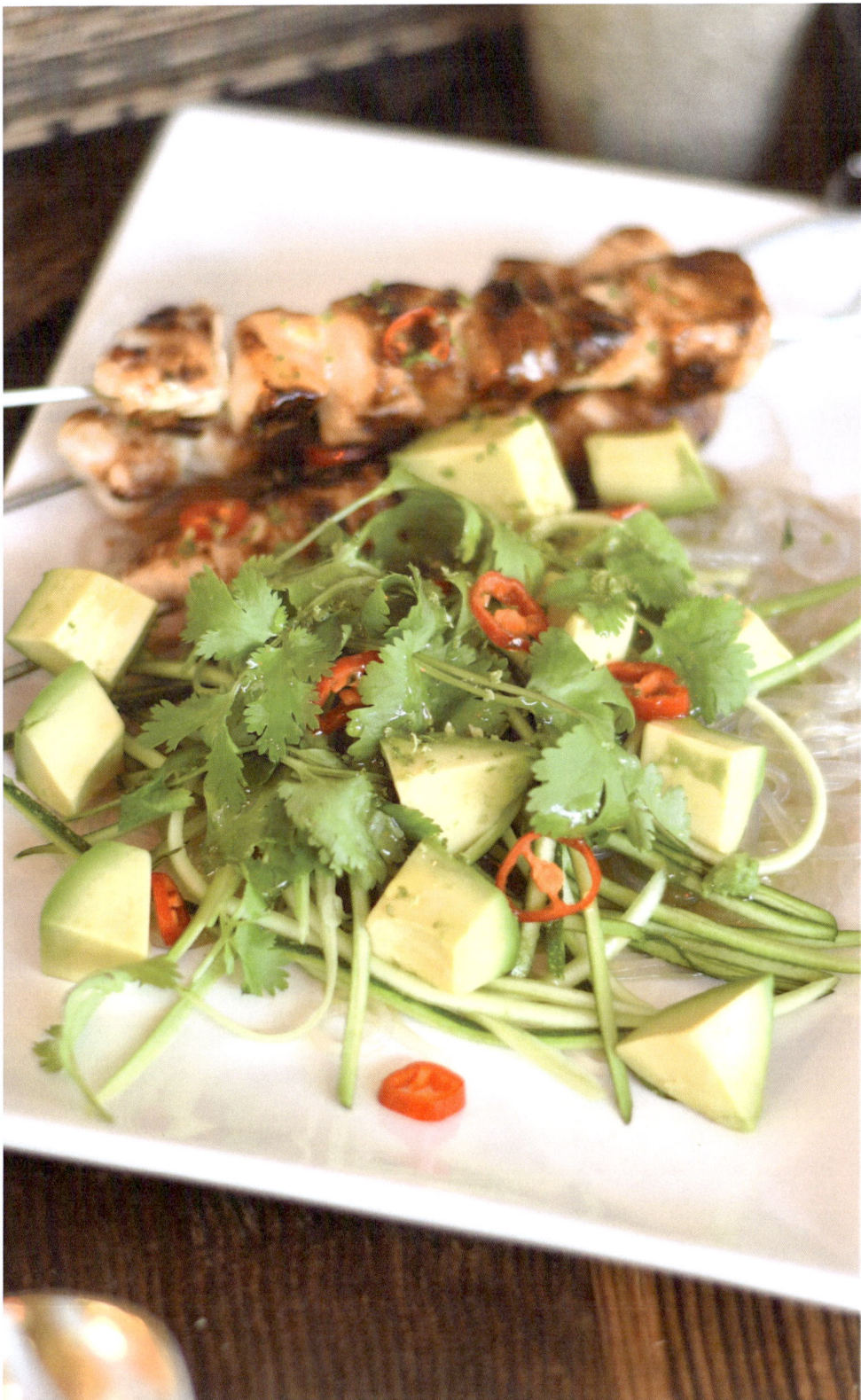

WELLBEING
Connect with Nature

Many studies confirm a direct connection to nature is essential for our health and wellbeing.[1] We are happier and less stressed when we spend significant time in nature. Our relationships are healthier, we are more self-confident and are much more physically healthy after spending time outdoors.

The feeling of bliss and relaxation you get when you venture into the great outdoors has a lot of science supporting it. Breathing in fresh air benefits the lungs and brain and contributes to a sense of wellbeing. This works because fresh, clean air regulates serotonin and melatonin levels. The negative iron-rich oxygen also relaxes the body. Vitamin D is produced by our bodies when exposed to sunshine and improves blood flow and blood pressure and relaxes the blood vessels.

Merely disconnecting from work, emails and phones allow us to relax fully. Outdoor activities (including gardening) are excellent at reducing our stress levels. Our stress hormone levels drop and our mood improves when we're outside in nature. Deeper breathing stimulates the body's parasympathetic reaction calming us down and reducing stress.

The physical nature of being outside means you're exercising more and this releases endorphins (the feel-good neurotransmitters) helping us feel clear-headed, calm and relaxed.

- Switch off from your busy worklife, emails and phones

- Connect deeply with nature ~ walk, hike, run or simply spend time outdoors

- Breathe deeply ~ consciously/ meditatively

- Fresh air regulates serotonin and melatonin improving mood and concentration

- Vitamin D enhances blood flow and pressure and relaxes the blood vessels

- Breathing deeply stimulates the parasympathetic system calming us down

- Being active outdoors releases 'feel good' endorphins

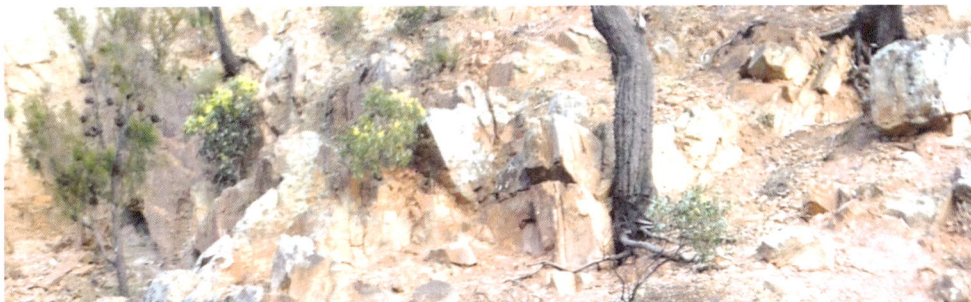

*Look deep into nature, and then you
will understand everything better*

Albert Einstein

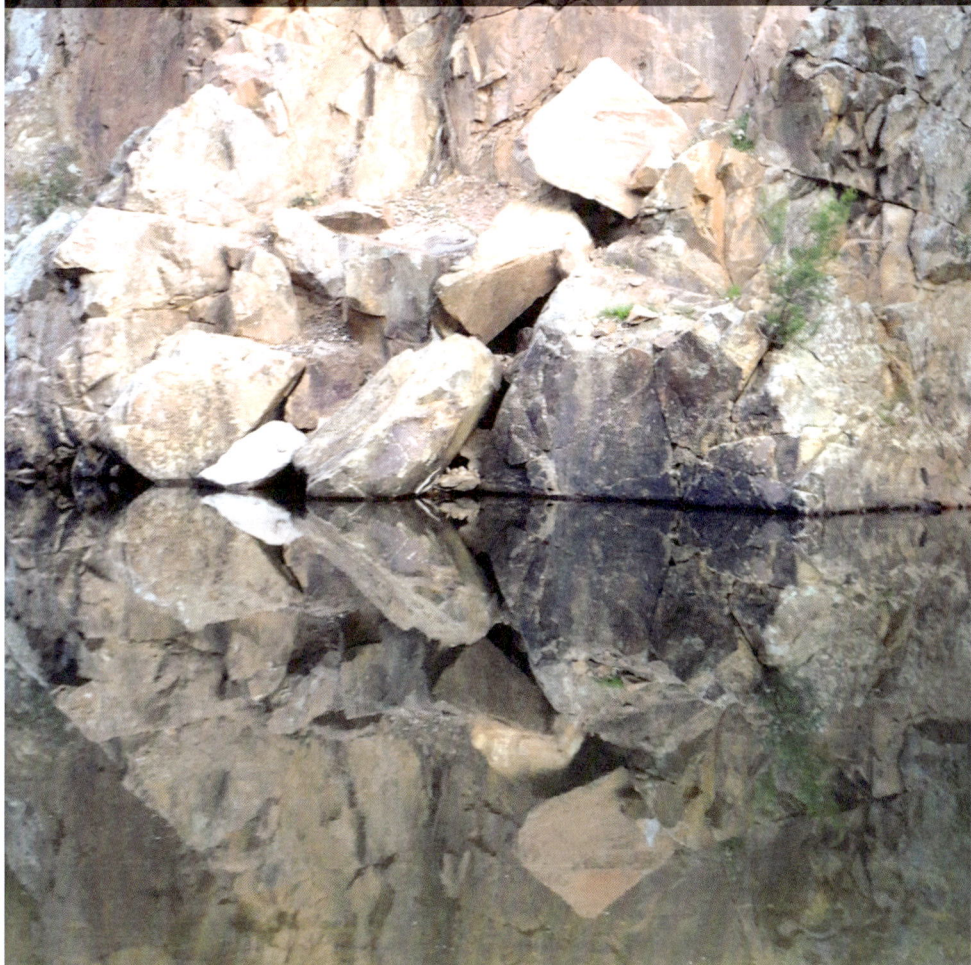

Yoga

Originating in ancient India, yoga offers a comprehensive approach by seamlessly combining powerful physical, mental, and spiritual practices.

It treats the mind and body as an integrated system, fostering self-regulation across physical, mental, and emotional dimensions, establishing itself as a therapeutic discipline through extensive research[1-2].

The mental health benefits of yoga are intricately linked to the vagus nerve, leading to significant reductions in stress, anxiety, fatigue, and depression[3-4].

Beyond mental well-being, yoga contributes to lower inflammation[5], improved heart health, better sleep, and an overall enhanced quality of life. Notably, its efficacy extends to alleviating chronic pain symptoms, concurrently promoting flexibility, balance, and improved breathing. The integration of yogic concepts like mindful eating further amplifies its impact, supporting optimal body functions, effective weight management, and the development of healthier habits.

This holistic practice, born from ancient wisdom, emerges as a powerful and multifaceted approach to overall well-being[6].

Meditation and Mindfulness

Meditation and mindfulness have many powerful health benefits including calming the mind and reducing stress, anxiety and depression.[1] Meditation increases self-awareness, kindness, attention span, controls pain and can even decrease your blood pressure. "Structural and functional brain changes have been demonstrated in the brains of people with a long-term traditional meditation practice, and in people who have completed a MBSR [mindfulness-based stress reduction] programme."[2] Mindfulness exercises help you get into 'the flow' where you are in a beautiful and calm state of mind. Simple things such as colouring in for five minutes daily can relax and soothe our nerves. It lowers our blood pressure, can reduce chronic pain and allows our immune system to function efficiently.

Yesterday I was clever so I wanted to change the world. Today I am wise so I am changing myself

Rumi

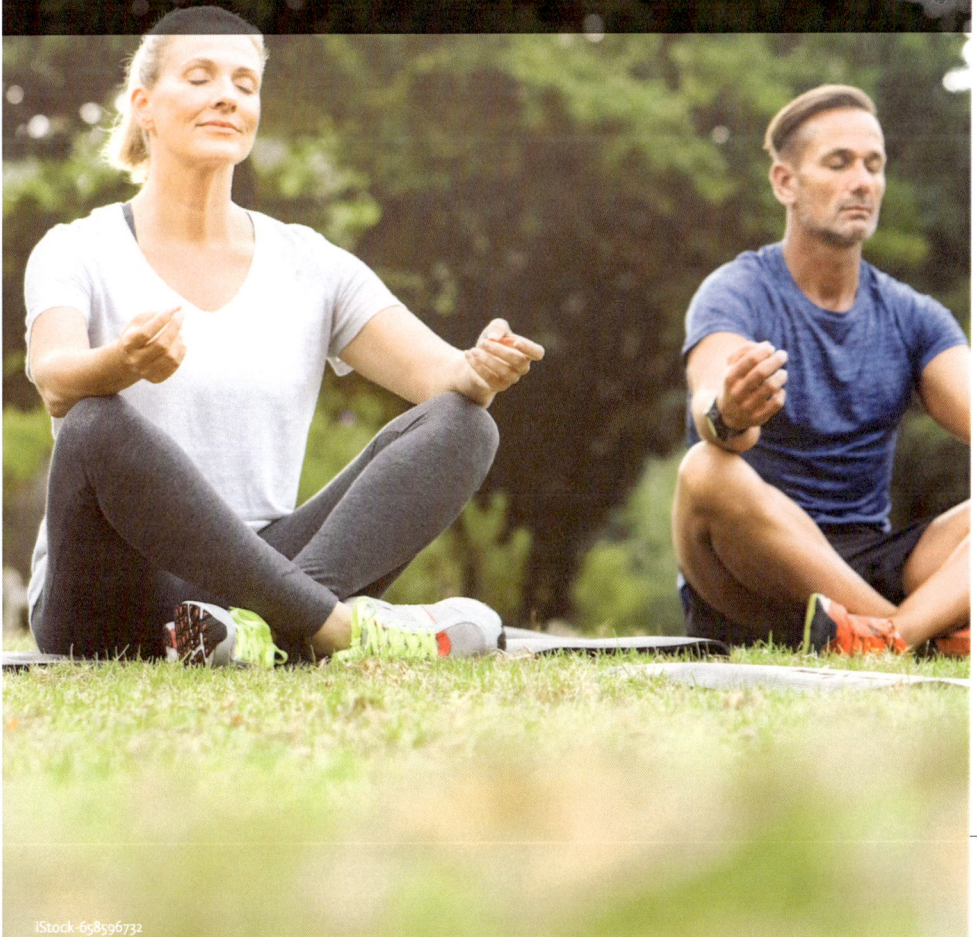

You cannot always control what goes on outside.
But you can always control what goes on inside

Wayne Dyer

iStock-658596732

I've been studying happiness for 20 years and it turns out it's simple. Find awe

Prof Dacher Keltner, University of California, Berkeley

Awe Hunting

Awe hunting encourages us to actively seek moments of profound wonder in our daily lives. Dacher Keltner, a renowned professor of psychology at the University of California and author of "Awe: The New Science of Everyday Wonder and How It Can Transform Your Life," champions the value of pursuing awe-inspiring experiences. Engaging in awe hunting connects us to the world on a profound level, fostering personal growth, mental well-being and a profound sense of purpose[1].

Keltner's research illustrates that awe has a transformative power, expanding our perspective and reinforcing our place within the vast cosmos. Whether it's gazing at a star-studded night sky or standing before a majestic waterfall, awe inspires humility and a heightened sense of interconnectedness.

Keltner aptly observes, "Awe is the ultimate integrative emotion, bringing people together, fostering tolerance, cooperation, and positive social emotions." Awe transcends divisions, facilitating empathy and building communities. In today's divided world, this is especially significant.

Julia Baird, an accomplished Australian journalist, also underscores the significance of awe. She aptly notes, "Awe stops time and shrinks our ego, allowing us to tap into something larger than ourselves."

Awe hunting offers a welcome escape from the stresses of daily life, immersing us in a timeless state of pure appreciation, momentarily releasing the burdens of the ego.

Furthermore, awe has been scientifically linked to various mental and emotional benefits, including stress reduction, increased well-being, and heightened creativity. It also instills a greater sense of purpose in life. Actively seeking opportunities for awe hunting enriches our lives, leading to greater happiness and fulfillment.

Awe hunting inspires us to actively seek out moments of wonder and amazement in our lives. As Dacher Keltner and Julia Baird emphasise, these awe-filled experiences connect us to the world, foster unity, and enhance our overall well-being. Awe hunting isn't just a leisurely pursuit; it's a transformative practice that can lead to a more meaningful and satisfying life. By actively seeking awe-inspiring experiences, we tap into the profound benefits of wonder and, in the process, become more compassionate, connected and inspired individuals.

The Vagus Nerve

Stimulating the vagus nerve significantly enhances both physical and mental well-being. This intricate nerve connects to vital organs like the heart, lungs, and digestive system, playing a crucial role in regulating essential bodily functions.[1-2] Activating the vagus nerve brings numerous health benefits, elevating the overall quality of life.

One notable advantage of vagus nerve stimulation is its swift reduction of stress by initiating the body's "rest and digest" response, countering the typical "fight or flight" stress reaction. This, in turn, leads to a decrease in cortisol levels and anxiety. Simple practices like deep breathing exercises and mindfulness meditation effectively engage the vagus nerve, inducing a state of relaxation.

Moreover, the vagus nerve has a significant impact on heart health by regulating heart rate, maintaining a steady rhythm, and reducing the risk of heart disease. Techniques such as slow, deep breathing contribute to lowering heart rate and blood pressure, promoting long-term cardiovascular well-being.

The vagus nerve also plays a crucial role in enhancing digestion by increasing stomach acid secretion and promoting peristalsis, aiding nutrient absorption and alleviating digestive discomfort, including symptoms of irritable bowel syndrome (IBS).

Effective methods for vagus nerve stimulation encompass various practices such as deep breathing exercises, mindfulness meditation, yoga, cold exposure, vocalization activities like singing or humming, gargling, and maintaining social connections. These activities engage the vagus nerve's calming "rest and digest" response, promoting relaxation, reducing stress, and improving mental health.[3-4]

Whether through deep breaths or shared laughter with friends, regular engagement with these techniques can unlock the vagus nerve's potential for holistic well-being.

In a broader context, evidence suggests that stimulating the vagus nerve may play a role in slowing tumor development through its anti-inflammatory effects on the body's immune responses, potentially improving outcomes for cancer patients.[5]

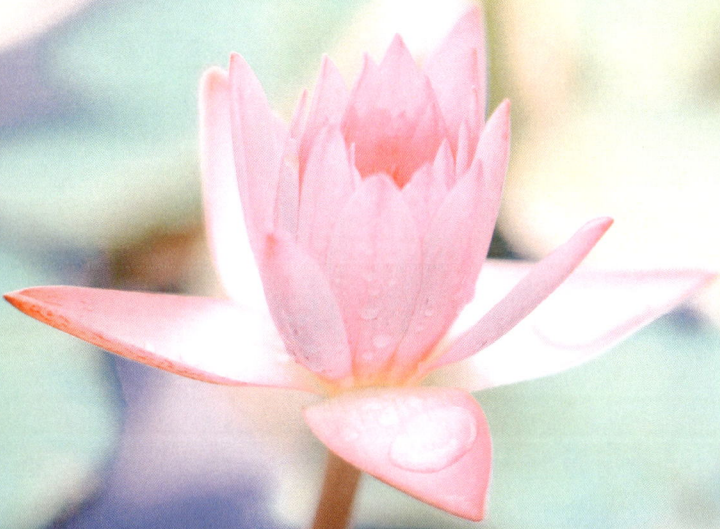

Let the breath lead the way

Sharon Salzberg

Time doesn't heal emotional pain,
you need to learn how to let go

Roy Bennett

Releasing Suppressed Emotions

Perhaps one of the most important ways to heal from cancer is to release suppressed emotions.[1] Emotional trauma and intense emotions such as extreme stress, anger, fear, resentment and anxiety can create embedded tension in our body and damages our DNA.[2] Stress is our body's natural response to difficulties or pressure. The body releases stress hormones including adrenaline and cortisol and readies your body for fight or flight. A prolonged state of stress from unresolved emotions may lead to disease and cancer.[3] Often cancer patients can point to a significantly stressful event six months to two years before their cancer diagnosis.

The first step and perhaps the most effective way to start releasing these emotions is to talk about them, face them and begin to accept them. Opening up to a close friend or talking with a psychotherapist/counsellor are great options. You can consider daily forgiveness practices. You could write letters detailing your trauma or other emotional events and burn them rather than send them to anyone. Other options include guided imagery[4], energy healing[5], Eye Movement Desensitisation and Reprocessing (EMDR)[6] and Emotional Freedom Technique (EFT)[7] also referred to as tapping. Working with a professional may give you the best long term results.

Daily Forgiveness and Gratitude

You could practice a simple mantra each day such as 'I'm ok, I forgive myself, I forgive others'. Gratitude strategies, applied daily, will improve mental well-being, enhance relationships, and foster positivity.

Energy Healing

Reiki means 'universal life energy'. It's a gentle therapy using energy fields in and around the body. Practitioners transfer universal energy through 'palm healing' and help restore emotional and physical health.

Emotional Freedom Technique (EFT)

EFT, or tapping, focuses on meridian or energy points in the body. It draws on various practices including acupuncture, neuro-linguistic programming, energy medicine, and Thought Field Therapy. It restores energy balance and relieves negative emotions.

LONG TERM

Holistic Health

You now know what to do each day and how to maintain that approach over the long term. It's a challenging journey so don't be too hard on yourself if you're not perfect along the way. There will be plenty of bumps and you'll probably fall off the wagon at times. Dust yourself off and get back on track. The best advice is to keep going and focus on your long term healing goal. In some respects it's like training and running a marathon. It takes a lot of time but absolutely anyone can do it if they train carefully and work at it.

Test and monitor

The way you feel will probably be the best guide to how you are actually going. If you're following all of these suggested guidelines you will gradually (maybe very quickly) start to feel better and much more in control of where things are going. Some people feel reassured by having regular blood tests to ensure that the process you are working through is right for your body and your illness. Some people find that takes their focus away from their positive new lifestyle but others like that reassurance that things are going well.

I think it's wise to keep an eye on things with testing. That will also reassure others you're on the right track. All cancers are different and may respond very differently so take care and don't just assume everything is perfect. Be sure. If you need to reduce stress more then focus on that. If you think you need a short fast to rebalance and give your digestive system a rest, do that carefully so you don't lose much weight.

Continue to empower yourself

Keep researching and learning about new approaches so you can adjust as new science emerges. It takes many years for the new ideas to make their way into the mainstream medical fields so maintain your knowledge.

Keep going

It will be a long journey so pace yourself and try to maintain a lifestyle that you can continue. Burn out is a risk so try to build those daily habits and ask others to help you.

You've got this.

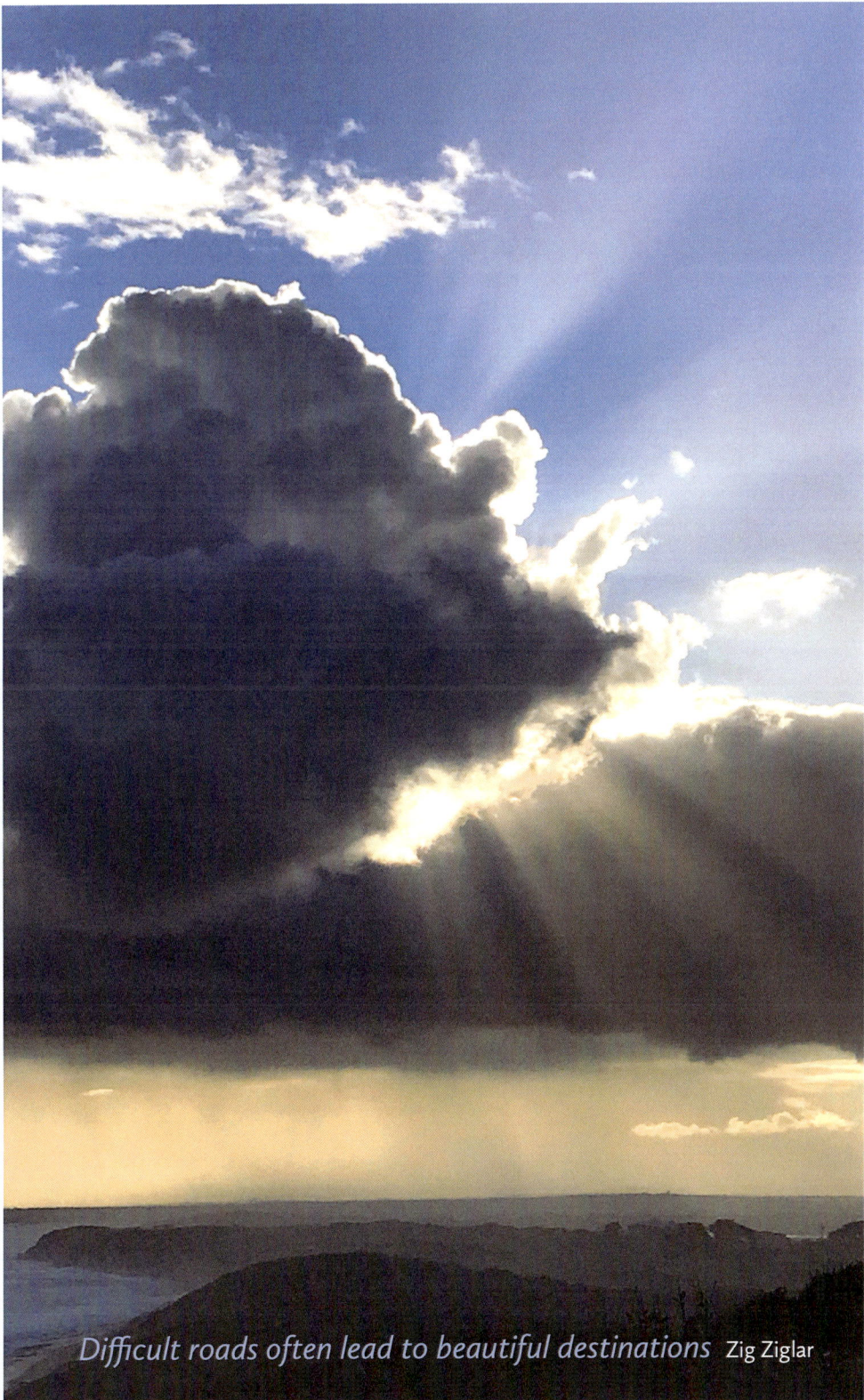

Difficult roads often lead to beautiful destinations Zig Ziglar

The world breaks everyone,
and afterward many are strong at the broken places

Ernest Hemingway

MANAGING AND SURVIVING *Cancer*

A cancer journey is a life-changing experience. Managing and surviving cancer can have a different meaning for different people. Some might be successfully managing their treatment and symptoms on a long term basis. Others may have survived cancer and be completely free from cancer signs. Wherever you are on that journey, you may experience some deep emotions about how you got to where you are, why you've managed or survived and others perhaps have not and where you go from here.

Feeling guilt and fear

Some people feel guilty about their positive outcome and perhaps feel they don't deserve or didn't work hard enough to achieve it or someone else who didn't survive should have. Whatever thoughts you have, please be reassured it's not your fault. It's a complex journey and whatever has happened in the past is best accepted and left there. It can be a fearful time not knowing if you'll remain cancer-free. Increasing positive emotions is an important focus to manage and maintain a balance as a survivor.

Whichever way you view it you need to adjust to the new space. This may mean accepting some changes to the way you live or look after yourself. It may take you a while to rebalance completely and feel positive and grateful for your journey. That's ok. Take your time. If you need assistance don't hesitate to ask for help or seek counselling support. It's a challenging journey and we all need a little help now and again.

Rediscover yourself

Some people rediscover a zest for life and rediscover more meaningful relationships. Some reassess their careers and make significant changes. Some broaden their horizons and travel or get involved in new hobbies. Some find meaning in helping others through their healing journey.

- Whatever you do, relax and accept it will be ok

- Let go of how you got here and realise you've done your best

- Find that zest for life, your ecstasy, and keep on going

PREPARING
For All Outcomes

The reality is, cancer is a complex and life-threatening range of diseases and healing is a difficult journey. You may have heard the saying "prepare for the worst but expect the best". It means carefully assessing what may happen and preparing for that just in case but aiming for and expecting the best outcome. Being prepared will help you stay focussed. If things take a turn for the worst it can happen very quickly and can be overwhelming. If you haven't sat down with your loved ones before then to discuss all of the possibilities, it just adds more pressure and stress to deal with it and cope with the progressing disease.

It makes sense to sort through a lot of the challenging issues well and truly beforehand to enable you to focus on getting better. It is very difficult to contemplate the possibility of dying, either from the point of view of the cancer patient, or of family and loved ones, but avoiding this discussion is unfortunately, at times, avoiding an inevitable event.

These are some of the tough conversations that you may want to have:

- Update your will, superannuation beneficiaries and other financial matters

- Include specific requests for burial or cremation etc.

- Include details about who will get each of your main assets, possessions etc (consider pets)

- Sort out any insurance or other legal concerns

- Try to tidy up your things to reduce any complexities and points of contention should you pass away

- Talk to each of your family and friends about your requests so it's clear to all concerned

- If required, organise 'Voluntary Assisted Dying' or similar needs with your medical support team. This can be a lengthy process so get started early if possible, just in case it is needed.

Prepare for the worst but...
EXPECT the best

iStock_000025689510

Only in the darkness can you see the stars Martin Luther King Jr

93

ADVANCED CANCER ~ Cachexia
Your Body Can Still Heal

Cachexia a wasting disorder which affects up to 80% of late stage cancer patients. About one-third of these patients die of complications relating to this condition. Cachexia is a combination of Systemic inflammation, gut dysfunction and extreme muscle loss. Systemic inflammation may be a direct result of cancer or the body's reaction to the tumour. As the body's immune system is overwhelmed gut dysfunction increases.
Good bacteria in the gut, such as lactobacillus are wiped out allowing inflammation-causing bacteria to flourish. The overall result is often rapid decline with overwhelming symptoms and death, sometimes occurring extremely fast, in a matter of days or weeks.

Conventional approaches focus on easing symptoms and providing comfort as the disease advances. Emerging research indicates you may be able to reverse this process and heal.

Late Stage Symptoms

- Increased pain
- High calcium levels (can be prognostic and/or causal)
- Confusion, leading to poor choices
- Nausea
- Gut dysfunction poor digestion and wrong feelings of fullness
- Fatigue
- Cachexia (rapid skeletal muscle loss)
- Constipation

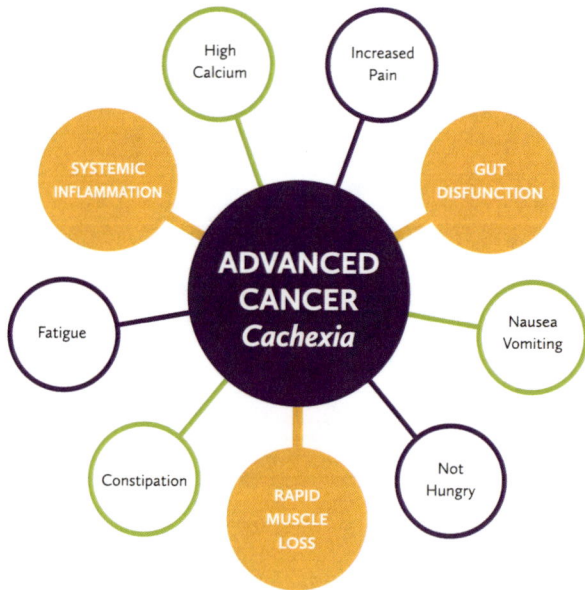

CACHEXIA ~ Triggers

Early Detection is Essential

Advanced cancer is when tumours dramatically increase in size or spread throughout the body. They release substances that reduce our appetite. Some treatments can also cause severe nausea or damage the digestive system making it difficult to eat. As the body gets fewer nutrients, it burns fat and muscle to support the brain. Inflammation and pain increase, high calcium levels lead to confusion, nausea and fatigue.

The digestive system may stop working and can cause constipation. This can all occur in a matter of days or weeks.

Early cachexia can be detected, and emerging research indicates it may be stopped and reversed. Cachexia can be detected early through regular mid-upper arm muscle measurements and blood tests.

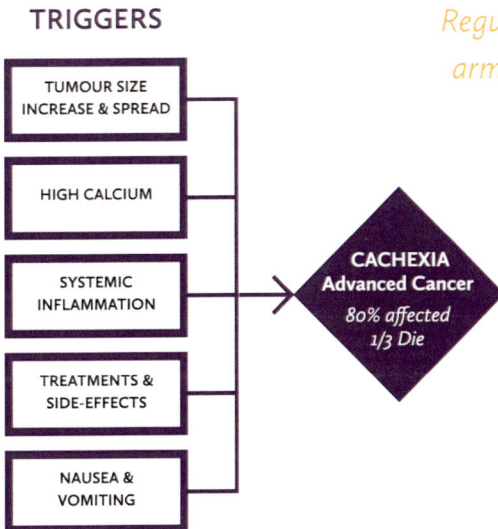

TRIGGERS

Regularly measure mid-upper arm muscle area (MUAMA)

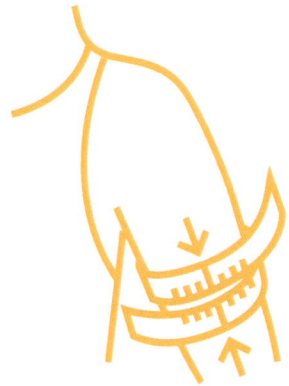

TUMOUR SIZE
INCREASE & SPREAD

HIGH CALCIUM

SYSTEMIC
INFLAMMATION

TREATMENTS &
SIDE-EFFECTS

NAUSEA &
VOMITING

CACHEXIA
Advanced Cancer
80% affected
1/3 Die

STOP & REVERSE CACHEXIA
Rebalance the Microbiome

Fecal Microbiota Transplant & Intravenous Vitamin C

Emerging research suggests that the body may have the potential to rebalance and heal even in the late stages; however, once cachexia becomes too advanced, halting its progression becomes extremely challenging. Reversing systemic inflammation, a significant factor in cachexia, shows promise with key interventions, including Fecal Microbiota Transplant (FMT)[1-2-3-4] and Intravenous Vitamin C (IVC)[5-6]. Using these safe treatments may require insistence, as current practitioners are likely to downgrade or ridicule their effectiveness. Desperate times call for desperate measures!

Fecal Microbiota Transplant involves transferring healthy donor fecal microbiota into the intestine of a cancer patient, aiming to restore gut flora balance and reduce inflammation.

Intravenous Vitamin C, administered directly into the bloodstream, exhibits anti-inflammatory properties by modulating immune responses and neutralising free radicals. IVC, recognised as a safe treatment, has shown effectiveness in reversing sepsis and holds potential for treating cancer cachexia.

Other Strategies

At this advanced stage, though the effectiveness of these strategies may be limited, any additional improvement can contribute to a successful rebalance. Strategies include increasing pre and probiotics, engaging in exercise[7], de-stressing, and stimulating your vagus nerve[8] to counteract systemic inflammation, gut dysfunction, and skeletal muscle loss. Prebiotics and probiotics play a crucial role in fostering a healthy gut microbiome, while exercise, including specific activities like sit-to-stands, push-ups, and weight training, has been shown to reduce inflammation and benefit the immune system.

De-stressing through activities like meditation, yoga and walking helps to stimulate your vagus nerve and further aids in reducing inflammation and improving overall well-being. Addressing electrolyte imbalances induced by constant vomiting is crucial, with options such as coconut water or electrolyte drinks for minor imbalances, along with close monitoring by caregivers. Elevated calcium levels can impact cognitive function, necessitating fluid therapy. Early intervention is critical for successful management, emphasising the importance of vigilant patient monitoring and promptly seeking medical attention.

Early Intervention is Crucial to Success

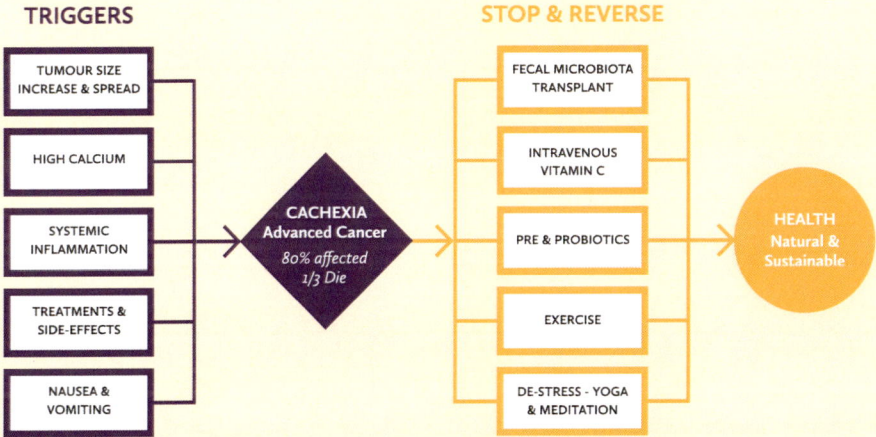

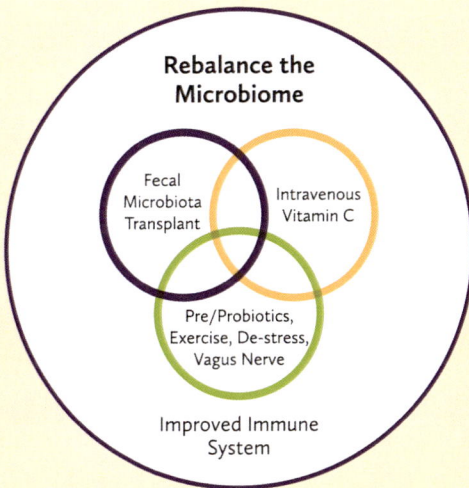

TRIGGERS

- TUMOUR SIZE INCREASE & SPREAD
- HIGH CALCIUM
- SYSTEMIC INFLAMMATION
- TREATMENTS & SIDE-EFFECTS
- NAUSEA & VOMITING

CACHEXIA
Advanced Cancer
80% affected
1/3 Die

STOP & REVERSE

- FECAL MICROBIOTA TRANSPLANT
- INTRAVENOUS VITAMIN C
- PRE & PROBIOTICS
- EXERCISE
- DE-STRESS - YOGA & MEDITATION

HEALTH
Natural &
Sustainable

Rebalance the Microbiome

Fecal Microbiota Transplant

Intravenous Vitamin C

Pre/Probiotics, Exercise, De-stress, Vagus Nerve

Improved Immune System

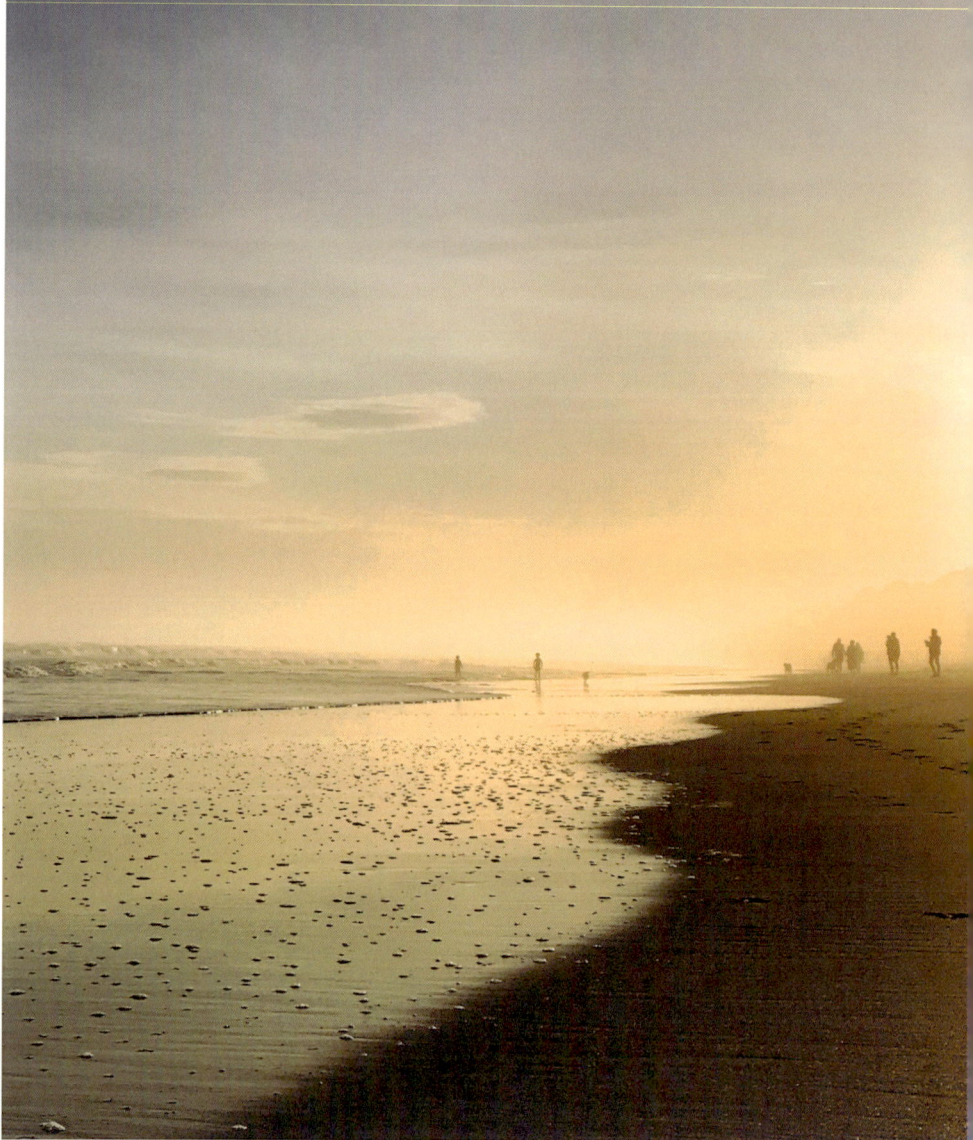

It's not what happens to you,
but how you react that matters

Epictetus

SAYING GOODBYE
Grief and Loss

All things must eventually pass. It's the natural way. If you've tried everything and things still aren't improving it may be time to say goodbye. It's very important to remember that you haven't failed, it's just that the cancer is complex. These things are sometimes beyond our control and we have to accept that we've tried our best and that's ok. That in itself is a beautiful and remarkable thing. Don't give up but start to make preparations.

At some point you may become very sick and unable to communicate with your loved ones. While you have time, it's best to tell them how much you love them and to say goodbye. It's incredibly difficult. You may not want to give in and that's commendable but please prepare and say farewell anyhow. You may miss the opportunity to speak to those closest to you.

Some people take the time to write letters to their loved ones to say things they perhaps have meant to say for a long time or to say things that are difficult to say face to face. These letters can then be treasured memories to help those left behind. These will help them get through.

- You haven't failed. You've tried your best and that's ok

- Don't give up. Keep trying to stop and reverse cachexia by following the steps in the previous pages

- Ask your loved ones to be close by. Sharing this time is truly special

- Ask others for extra assistance if needed

- Say goodbyes sooner rather than later

As a carer, you've been very involved in supporting your loved one through this long and challenging journey. If your loved one dies your grief can be overwhelming and hard to understand. Grief is different for everyone. You may experience it in waves even before your loved one passes away. Realising there's nothing you can do to help or save them is devastating. The process of dealing with the pain of loss and letting go is exceptionally hard and will take time to deal with. Don't be too hard on yourself if your emotions are unpredictable. It's ok. Try to be kind and considerate to others. Your pain will ease with time.

CARING FOR SOMEONE
With Cancer

Caring for a loved one or friend as they journey through cancer is challenging. You need to care for yourself in the process to ensure you can keep looking after them. Like the 'oxygen mask on the plane situation', you need to look after yourself first to then look after others. If you can attend medical appointments with them, take notes, ask questions and discuss things afterwards that will be a great help as long as this is what they want. You may need to reduce your workload to look after them. This is temporary and worth putting in extra effort to help them along the way particularly in the early stages as they grapple with all of the dimensions of their diagnosis and disease. Try to remain calm and positive and follow this guide in previous chapters. Empower the patient as much as possible.

- Support the patient's approach even if you disagree. Explain why you disagree but support their decisions

- Assist with medical appointments, take notes and be a good listener and sounding board

- Support them by researching as much as possible too

Sometimes there are multiple complications and the patient can become very sick. This can happen very quickly. Caring for someone as they die is perhaps the greatest privilege. They are entrusting their total care to you. That's incredibly significant and can weigh heavily on you. You may feel you could have done things differently or feel responsible somehow. It's not your fault and be reassurred you haven't failed. It's a complicated and long journey and sometimes not everything goes right. It's ok. Being grateful for the beautiful things is challenging but essential to finding a long term balance. Focusing on the wonderful memories is important for your healing and to enable you to let go and move on.

- Be kind to each other. You're all going through incredibly difficult times

- Get assistance if your emotions are out of balance and you feel it's too difficult to manage

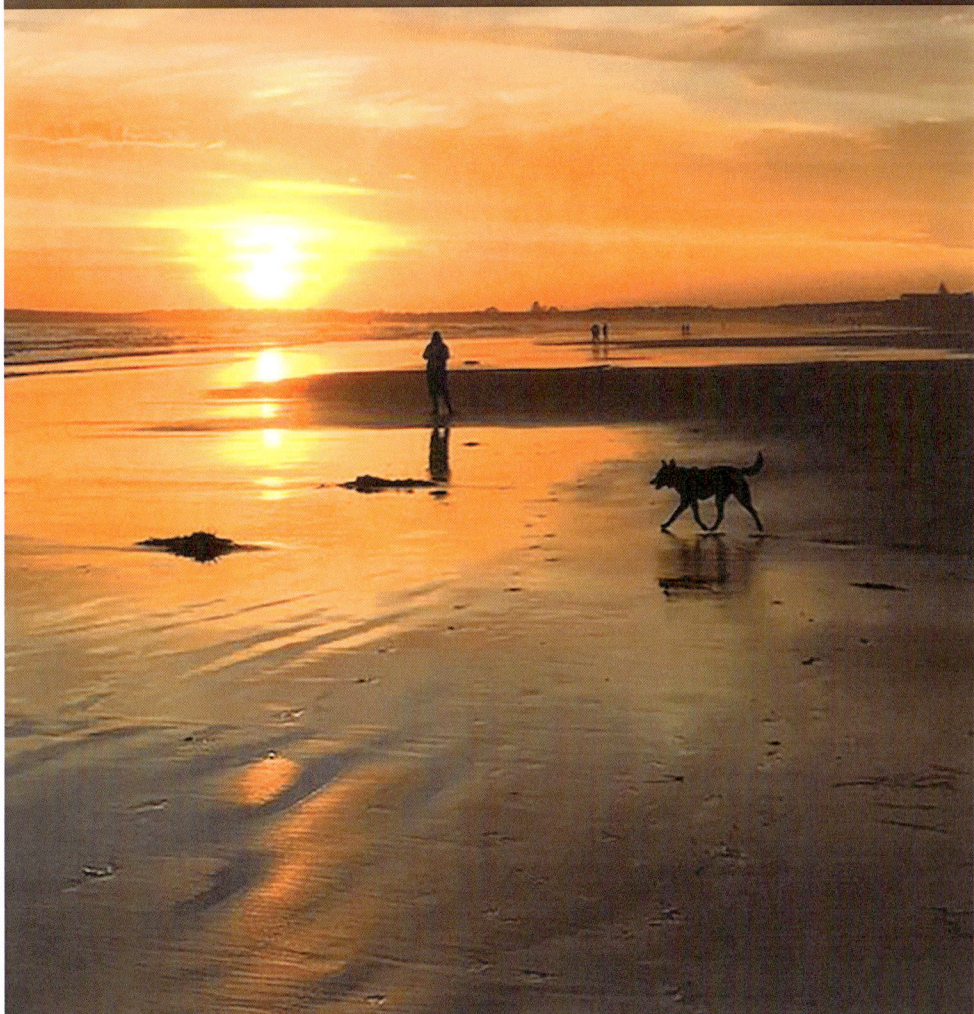

Life is like riding a bicycle.
To keep your balance you must keep moving

Albert Einstein, letter to his son Eduard, 1930

Don't ever
Give up hope!

Tomorrow... repeat

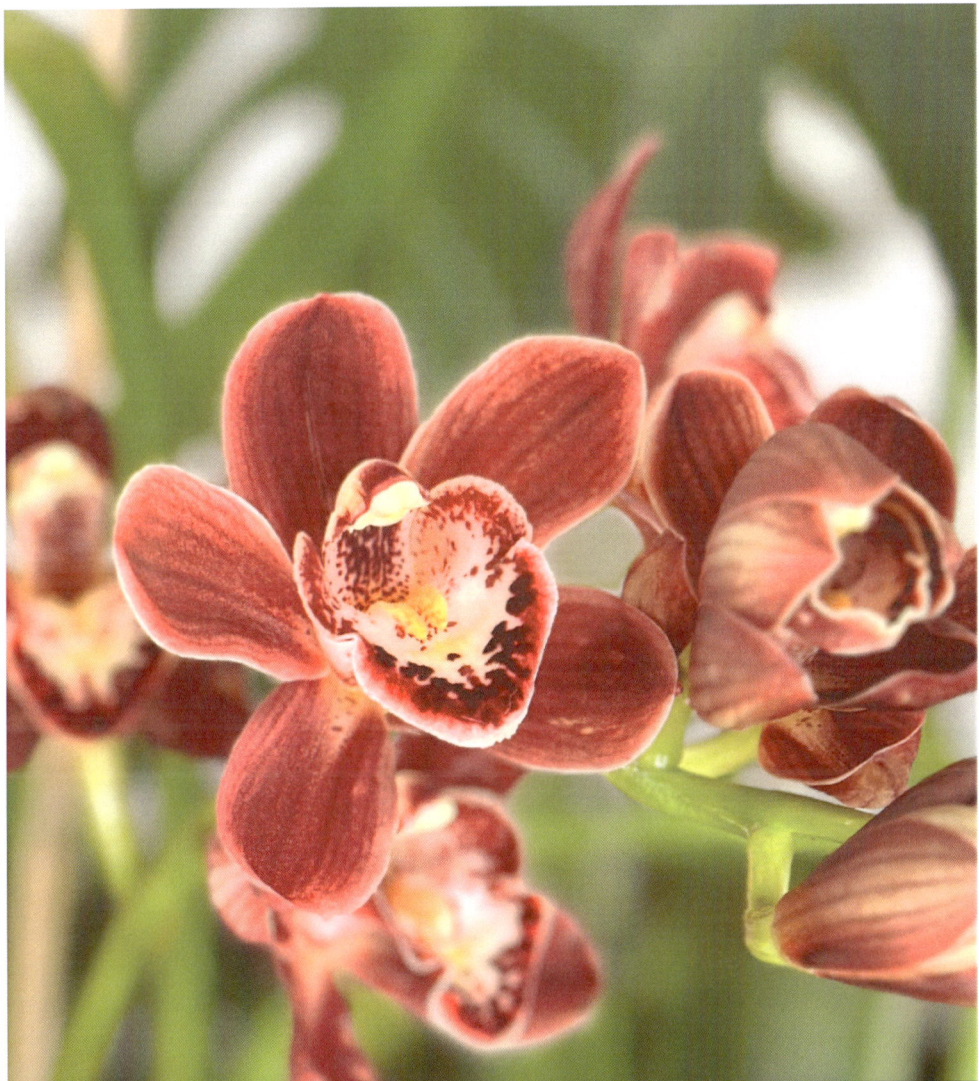

Be the change you wish to see in the world

Mahatma Gandhi

REFERENCES

Chapter 2 - So you have cancer

1   Deleemans, J. M., et al. "The chemo-gut study: investigating the long-term effects of chemotherapy on gut microbiota, metabolic, immune, psychological and cognitive parameters in young adult Cancer survivors; study protocol". December 2019. BMC Cancer 19(1). DOI: 10.1186/s12885-019-6473-8. https://www.researchgate.net/publication/338121426_The_chemo-gut_study_investigating_the_long-term_effects_of_chemotherapy_on_gut_microbiota_metabolic_immune_psychological_and_cognitive_parameters_in_young_adult_Cancer_survivors_study_protocol

2   Konstantinidis, T., et al. "Effects of Antibiotics upon the Gut Microbiome: A Review of the Literature". Published online 2020 Nov 16. doi: 10.3390/biomedicines8110502. https://www.ncbi.nlm.nih.gov/pmc/articles/PMC7696078/

3   Weaver, KE., et al. "Mental and physical health-related quality of life among U.S. cancer survivors: population estimates from the 2010 National Health Interview Survey. 21 November 2012. https://pubmed.ncbi.nlm.nih.gov/23112268/#:~:text=Results%3A%20Poor%2physical%20and%20mental,poor%2physical%20and%20mental%20HRQOL.

4   Firkins, J. et al. "Quality of life in "chronic" cancer survivors: a meta-analysis." 11 March 2020. https://link.springer.com/article/10.1007/s11764-020-00869-9

5   Iddir. M., et al. "Strengthening the Immune System and Reducing Inflammation and Oxidative Stress through Diet and Nutrition: Considerations during the COVID-19 Crisis". Published online 2020 May 27. doi: 10.3390/nu12061562. https://www.ncbi.nlm.nih.gov/pmc/articles/PMC7352291/

6   Kouakanou, L. et al. "Vitamin C, From Supplement to Treatment: A Re-Emerging Adjunct for Cancer Immunotherapy?". 12 November 2021. https://www.frontiersin.org/articles/10.3389/fimmu.2021.765906/full

7   Baruch, E.N. et al. "Fecal microbiota transplant promotes response in immunotherapy-refractory melanoma patients". 10 December 2020. https://www.science.org/doi/10.1126/science.abb5920

Chapter 3 - Holistic approaches

1   Fan, D., "Holistic integrative medicine: toward a new era of medical advancement". Published: 02 March 2017. https://pubmed.ncbi.nlm.nih.gov/28044221/

2   Kisling, L. A., "Alternative Medicine". July 27, 2020. https://www.ncbi.nlm.nih.gov/books/NBK538520/

Chapter 5 - IVC

1   Carr, A.C. Maggini, S. "Vitamin C and Immune Function." 3 November 2017. https://www.mdpi.com/2072-6643/9/11/1211

2   Kouakanou, L. Peters, C. Brown, C. E. Kabelitz, D. Wang, L. D. "Vitamin C, From Supplement to Treatment: A Re-Emerging Adjunct for Cancer Immunotherapy?". 12 November 2021. https://www.frontiersin.org/articles/10.3389/fimmu.2021.765906/full

3   Magrì, A. Germano, G. Lorenzato, A. Lamba, S. Chilà, R. Montone, M. Amodio, V. Ceruti, T. Sassi, F. Arena, S. Abrignani, S. D'Incalci, M. Zucchetti, M. Di Nicolantonio, F. Bardelli, A. "High-dose vitamin C enhances cancer immunotherapy." 26 February 2020. https://www.science.org/doi/10.1126/scitranslmed.aay8707

Chapter 6 - FMT

1   Baruch, E.N. Youngster, I. Ben-Betzalel, G. Ortenberg, R. Lahat, A. Katz, L. Adler, K. Dick-Necula, D. Raskin, S. Bloch, N. Rotin, D. Anafi, L. Avivi, C. Melnichenko, J. Steinberg-Silman, Y. Mamtani,R. Harati, H. Asher, N. Shapira-Frommer, R. Brosh-Nissimov, T. Eshet, Y. Ben-Simon, S. Ziv, O. Wadud Khan, M.A. Amit, M. Ajami, N.J. Barshack, I. Schachter, J. Wargo, J.A. Koren, O. Markel, G. Boursi, B. "Fecal microbiota transplant promotes response in immunotherapy-refractory melanoma patients". 10 December 2020. https://www.science.org/doi/10.1126/science.abb5920

2   McQuade, J. L. et al. "Gut microbiome modulation via fecal microbiota transplant to augment immunotherapy in patients with melanoma or other cancers." June 24, 2020. https://www.ncbi.nlm.nih.gov/pmc/articles/PMC7685568/

Chapter 7 -
Cancer Management Plan

1   Turner, J. et al. "Regular exercise has long-term benefits for immunity – it's important to stay active." April 10, 2020. https://theconversation.com/regular-exercise-has-long-term-benefits-for-immunity-its-important-to-stay-active-135836

2   Pascoe, M. "It's not all in your mind: how meditation affects the brain to help you stress less." August 22, 2018. https://theconversation.com/its-not-all-in-your-mind-how-meditation-affects-the-brain-to-help-you-stress-less-97777

3   Tang, Y. Y. et al. "Long-Term Physical Exercise and Mindfulness Practice in an Aging Population." April 2, 2020. https://www.ncbi.nlm.nih.gov/pmc/articles/PMC7142262/

4   Worthen, M. et al., "Stress Management". Last Update: August 29, 2020. https://www.ncbi.nlm.nih.gov/books/NBK513300/

5   Cormie P. "Every cancer patient should be prescribed exercise medicine". The Conversation, May 7, 2018. https://theconversation.com/every-cancer-patient-should-be-prescribed-exercise-medicine-95440

6   Chopra, D., "Deepak Chopra's 7-Step Exercise To Release Emotional Turbulence". Accessed January 15, 2021. https://www.gaiam.com/blogs/discover/deepak-chopras-7-step-exercise-to-release-emotional-turbulence#

7   Wahl, D. W., et al., "Healthy food choices are happy food choices: Evidence from a real life sample using smartphone based assessments". Published: 06 December 2017. https://www.nature.com/articles/s41598-017-17262-9

8   Gray, A., et al., "A review of nutrition and dietary interventions in oncology". Published online 2020 Jun 1. doi: 10.1177/2050312120926877. https://www.ncbi.nlm.nih.gov/pmc/articles/PMC7268120/

9   Kouakanou, L. Peters, C. Brown, C. E. Kabelitz, D. Wang, L. D. "Vitamin C, From Supplement to Treatment: A Re-Emerging Adjunct for Cancer Immunotherapy?". 12 November 2021. https://www.frontiersin.org/articles/10.3389/fimmu.2021.765906/full

10   Magrì, A. Germano, G. Lorenzato, A. Lamba, S. Chilà, R. Montone, M. Amodio, V. Ceruti, T. Sassi, F. Arena, S. Abrignani, S. D'Incalci, M. Zucchetti, M. Di Nicolantonio, F. Bardelli, A. "High-dose vitamin C enhances cancer immunotherapy." 26 February 2020. https://www.science.org/doi/10.1126/scitranslmed.aay8707

11   Morishita, S. et al., "Effect of Exercise on Mortality and Recurrence in Patients With Cancer: A Systematic Review and Meta-Analysis". Published online 2020 Jun 1. doi: 10.1177/1534735420917462. https://www.ncbi.nlm.nih.gov/pmc/articles/PMC7273753/

12   Chaudhury, P. et al., "Recovering With Nature: A Review of Ecotherapy and Implications for the COVID-19 Pandemic." Published online 2020 Dec 10. doi: 10.3389/fpubh.2020.604440. https://www.ncbi.nlm.nih.gov/pmc/articles/PMC7758313/

13   Bożek, A. et al., "The Relationship Between Spirituality, Health-Related Behavior, and Psychological Well-Being." Published online 2020 Aug 14. doi: 10.3389/fpsyg.2020.01997. https://www.ncbi.nlm.nih.gov/pmc/articles/PMC7457021/

14   Longo, V. "Nutrition and Fast-Mimicking Diet (FMD) for Cancer Prevention." Accessed January 15, 2021. https://www.valterlongo.com/cancer/

15   McQuade, J. L. et al. "Gut microbiome modulation via fecal microbiota transplant to augment immunotherapy in patients with melanoma or other cancers." June 24, 2020. https://www.ncbi.nlm.nih.gov/pmc/articles/PMC7685568/

Chapter 8 - Cancer

1   Cancer Australia. "Men's Health Week: Men more likely to develop and die from cancer". Release Date 17/06/2015. https://www.canceraustralia.gov.au/about-us/news/mens-health-week-men-more-likely-develop-and-die-cancer

2   Wu, S. et al., "Substantial contribution of extrinsic risk factors to cancer development." Published online 16 December 16, 2015. https://www.nature.com/articles/nature16166

3   Zhang, L., et al., "Chronic stress-induced immune dysregulation in cancer: implications for initiation, progression, metastasis, and treatment". Published online 2020 May 1. https://www.ncbi.nlm.nih.gov/pmc/articles/PMC7269780/

4   National Institute on Aging. "Research on intermittent fasting shows health benefits". February 27, 2020. https://www.nia.nih.gov/news/research-intermittent-fasting-shows-health-benefits

Chapter 9 - A Catalyst for Change

1   Turner, K. "Radical Hope - 10 Key Healing Factors from Exceptional Survivors of Cancer and other Diseases. April 2020

Chapter 11 - Brain-Gut - Communication

1   Sonnenburg, J. et al, "Gut Feelings - the "Second Brain" in Our Gastrointestinal Systems". May 1, 2015. https://www.scientificamerican.com/article/gut-feelings-the-second-brain-in-our-gastrointestinal-systems-excerpt/

2   Sullivan , E., "The Gut Health & Immunity Connection You Need To Know About, According To An MD. March 22, 2020. https://www.mindbodygreen.com/articles/the-probiotic-immunity-connection-this-md-wants-you-to-know-about

3   Deleemans, J. M., et al. "The chemo-gut study: investigating the long-term effects of chemotherapy on gut microbiota, metabolic, immune, psychological and cognitive parameters in young adult Cancer survivors; study protocol". December 2019. BMC Cancer 19(1). DOI: 10.1186/s12885-019-6473-8. https://www.researchgate.net/publication/338121426_The_chemo-gut_study_investigating_the_long-term_effects_of_chemotherapy_on_gut_microbiota_metabolic_immune_psychological_and_cognitive_parameters_in_young_adult_Cancer_survivors_study_protocol

4   Konstantinidis, T., et al. "Effects of Antibiotics upon the Gut Microbiome: A Review of the Literature". Published online 2020 Nov 16. doi: 10.3390/biomedicines8110502. https://www.ncbi.nlm.nih.gov/pmc/articles/PMC7696078/

5   Wang, J., et al. "Association between the gut microbiota and patient responses to cancer immune checkpoint inhibitors. December 2020. https://www.ncbi.nlm.nih.gov/pmc/articles/PMC7583737/

Chapter 12 -
The Immune System

1   Pandya, P. H. et al. "The Immune System in Cancer Pathogenesis: Potential Therapeutic Approaches." 2016 Dec 26. https://www.ncbi.nlm.nih.gov/pmc/articles/PMC5220497/

2   Zhang, L., et al., "Chronic stress-induced immune dysregulation in cancer: implications for initiation, progression, metastasis, and treatment". Published online 2020 May 1. https://www.ncbi.nlm.nih.gov/pmc/articles/PMC7269780/

Exercise

1   Cormie P. "Every cancer patient should be prescribed exercise medicine." The Conversation, May 7, 2018. https://theconversation.com/every-cancer-patient-should-be-prescribed-exercise-medicine-95440

2   Cormie P, et al. "The impact of exercise on cancer mortality, recurrence, and treatment-related adverse effects." Epidemiol Rev. 2017;39(1):71-92. https://www.ncbi.nlm.nih.gov/pubmed/28453622

3   Clinical Oncology Society of Australia. "COSA position statement on exercise in cancer care." April 2018. (update hyperlink to: https://www.cosa.org.au/media/332488/cosa-position-statement-v4-web-final.pdf

4   Clinical Oncology Society of Australia. Home page. Cited on September 19, 2018. from: https://www.cosa.org.au/

Nutrition

1   Soldati L, et al. "The influence of diet on anti-cancer immune responsiveness". 2018;20:3. https://www.ncbi.nlm.nih.gov/pmc/articles/PMC5859494/

2   Koutoukidis D, et al. "Lifestyle advice to cancer survivors: a qualitative study on the perspectives of health professionals." BMJ Open. 2018;8(3): e020313. https://www.ncbi.nlm.nih.gov/pmc/articles/PMC5875617/

3   Abrams, D. I. et al. "The cancer-fighting kitchen. Nourishing, big flavour recipes for cancer treatment and recovery." Katz, R. and Edelson, M. Authors. Second edition, 2017. Ten Speed Press, Berkeley. https://www.rebeccakatz.com/the-cancer-fighting-kitchen

4   Walia A. Ways Animal Protein Is Damaging Your Health. Collective-evolution. March 16, 2018. https://www.collective-evolution.com/2018/03/16/5-ways-animal-protein-is-damaging-your-health/

5   Morgan E. Levine, et al. Low Protein Intake is Associated with a Major Reduction in IGF-1, Cancer, and Overall Mortality in the 65 and Younger but Not Older Population. Cell Metab. 2014;4:3. https://www.ncbi.nlm.nih.gov/pmc/articles/PMC3988204/

Mediterranean & Ketogenic Diets

1   Schwingshacki L, et al. "Adherence to Mediterranean diet and risk of cancer: An updated systematic review and meta-analysis. Nutrients." 2017;9:10. https://www.ncbi.nlm.nih.gov/pmc/articles/PMC5691680/

2   Allen B, et al. "Ketogenic diets as an adjuvant cancer therapy: History and potential mechanism." 2014;7:8. https://www.ncbi.nlm.nih.gov/pmc/articles/PMC4215472/

3   Chung H, et al. "Rationale, Feasibility and Acceptability of Ketogenic Diet for Cancer Treatment." 2017;30:9. https://www.ncbi.nlm.nih.gov/pmc/articles/PMC5624453/

Herbs and Spices

1   Tomeh, M. A. et al. "A Review of Curcumin and Its Derivatives as Anticancer Agents." February 27, 2019. https://www.ncbi.nlm.nih.gov/pmc/articles/PMC6429287/

Teas

1   National Cancer Institute. "Tea and Cancer Prevention." Reviewed: November 17, 2010. https://www.cancer.gov/about-cancer/causes-prevention/risk/diet/tea-fact-sheet?redirect=true

Honey

2   Tahir AA, et al. "Combined ginger extract & Gelam honey modulate Ras/ERK and PI3K/AKT pathway genes in colon cancer HT29 cells." Nutr J. 2015;4:31. https://www.ncbi.nlm.nih.gov/pmc/articles/PMC4390091/

Chapter 16 - Wellbeing
Connect with Nature

1   Chaudhury, P. et al., "Recovering With Nature: A Review of Ecotherapy and Implications for the COVID-19 Pandemic." Published online 2020 Dec 10. doi: 10.3389/fpubh.2020.604440. https://www.ncbi.nlm.nih.gov/pmc/articles/PMC7758313/

Yoga

1   Syed S. et al. "A Brief Review of Beneficial Effects of Yoga on Physical and Mental Health." 29 August 2022. https://journal2.unusa.ac.id/index.php/MHSJ/article/view/3212

2   Büssing, A. et al. "Yoga as a Therapeutic Intervention." 11 November 2012. https://www.hindawi.com/journals/ecam/2012/174291/

3   Yoga for anxiety and depression". Harvard Mental Health Letter. Updated: October 13, 2020. https://www.health.harvard.edu/mind-and-mood/yoga-for-anxiety-and-depression

4   Syed S. et al. "A Brief Review of Beneficial Effects of Yoga on Physical and Mental Health." 29 August 2022. https://journal2.unusa.ac.id/index.php/MHSJ/article/view/3212

5   Yeun, Y.-R. et al. "Effects of yoga on immune function: A systematic review of randomized controlled trials." August 2021. https://www.sciencedirect.com/science/article/abs/pii/S1744388121001456?via%3Dihub

6   Madan, S. et al. "Yoga for Preventive Health: A Holistic Approach." 4 January 2022. https://journals.sagepub.com/doi/10.1177/15598276211059758

Meditation and Mindfulness

1   Sharma, H. "Meditation: Process and effects" 2015 July-September 2015. https://www.ncbi.nlm.nih.gov/pmc/articles/PMC4895748/

2   C. Behan, C. "The benefits of meditation and mindfulness practices during times of crisis such as COVID-19." May 14, 2020. https://www.ncbi.nlm.nih.gov/pmc/articles/PMC7287297/#

Awe Hunting

1   Yang Bai, Y. et al. "Awe, daily stress, and elevated life satisfaction." 1 April 2021. https://psycnet.apa.org/doiLanding?doi=10.1037%2Fpspa0000267

The Vagus Nerve

1   Larkin, T. "Our vagus nerves help us rest, digest and restore. Can you really reset them to feel better?" The Conversation. 24 August 2023. https://theconversation.com/our-vagus-nerves-help-us-rest-digest-and-restore-can-you-really-reset-them-to-feel-better-210469

2   Breit, S. Kupferberg, A. Rogler, G. Hasler, G. "Vagus Nerve as Modulator of the Brain–Gut Axis in Psychiatric and Inflammatory Disorders" 13 March 2018. https://www.frontiersin.org/articles/10.3389/fpsyt.2018.00044/full

3   Larkin, T. "Our vagus nerves help us rest, digest and restore. Can you really reset them to feel better?" The Conversation. 24 August 2023. https://theconversation.com/our-vagus-nerves-help-us-rest-digest-and-restore-can-you-really-reset-them-to-feel-better-210469

4   Trivedi, G. et al. "Humming (Simple Bhramari Pranayama) as a Stress Buster: A Holter-Based Study to Analyze Heart Rate Variability (HRV) Parameters During Bhramari, Physical Activity, Emotional Stress, and Sleep." 13 April 2023. https://www.ncbi.nlm.nih.gov/pmc/articles/PMC10182780/

5   Reijmen, E. Vannucci, L. De Couck, M. De Grève, J. Gidron, Y. "Therapeutic potential of the vagus nerve in cancer". 2 August 2018. https://www.sciencedirect.com/science/article/abs/pii/S0165247818301937?via%3Dihub

Releasing Suppressed Emotions

1   Chopra, D., "Deepak Chopra's 7-Step Exercise To Release Emotional Turbulence". Accessed January 15, 2021. https://www.gaiam.com/blogs/discover/deepak-chopras-7-step-exercise-to-release-emotional-turbulence#

2   Agnese Mariotti, A. "The effects of chronic stress on health: new insights into the molecular mechanisms of brain–body communication." November 2015. https://www.ncbi.nlm.nih.gov/pmc/articles/PMC5137920/

3   Slavich, G. M. "Life Stress and Health: A Review of Conceptual Issues and Recent Findings." August 16. 2016. https://www.ncbi.nlm.nih.gov/pmc/articles/PMC5066570/

4   Headspace. "Guided imagery". Accessed January 20, 2021. https://www.headspace.com/meditation/guided-imagery

5   Baron, M. et al. "What Everyone Should Know About Energy Healing." January 29, 2020. https://www.mindbodygreen.com/0-23890/what-everyone-should-know-about-energy-healing.html

6   American Psychological Association. "Eye Movement Desensitization and Reprocessing (EMDR) Therapy." Accessed January 20, 2021. https://www.apa.org/ptsd-guideline/treatments/eye-movement-reprocessing

7   Bach, D. et al. "Clinical EFT (Emotional Freedom Techniques) Improves Multiple Physiological Markers of Health." February 19, 2019. https://www.ncbi.nlm.nih.gov/pmc/articles/PMC6381429/

Chapter 19 -
Preparing for all Outcomes
Advanced Cancer ~ Cachexia

1   Panebianco, C. Villani, A. Potenza, A. Favaro, E. Finocchiaro, C. Perri, F. Pazienza, V. "Targeting Gut Microbiota in Cancer Cachexia: Towards New Treatment Options". 17 January 2023. https://www.mdpi.com/1422-0067/24/3/1849

2   Kelly M. , et al. "The Microbiota and Cancer Cachexia." December 2019. www.ncbi.nlm.nih.gov/pmc/articles/PMC6940781/#

3   Bindels, L. Neyrinck, A. Claus, S.P. Le Roy, C.L. Grangette, C. Pot, B Martínez, I. Walter, J. Cani, P.D. Delzenne, N. "Synbiotic approach restores intestinal homeostasis and prolongs survival in leukaemic mice with cachexia". 27 November 2015. https://www.nature.com/articles/ismej2015209

4   McQuade, J. L. et al. "Gut microbiome modulation via fecal microbiota transplant to augment immunotherapy in patients with melanoma or other cancers." June 24, 2020. https://www.ncbi.nlm.nih.gov/pmc/articles/PMC7685568/

5   Kashiouris, M. G. et al. "The Emerging Role of Vitamin C as a Treatment for Sepsis." January 22, 2020. https://www.ncbi.nlm.nih.gov/pmc/articles/PMC7070236/

6   Bindels, L. B. et al. "Nutrition in cancer patients with cachexia: A role for the gut microbiota?" April 2016. https://www.sciencedirect.com/science/article/pii/S2352939315000196

7   Daou, H. N. "Exercise as an anti-inflammatory therapy for cancer cachexia: a focus on interleukin-6 regulation." February 2020. https://pubmed.ncbi.nlm.nih.gov/31823669/

8   Breit, S. et al. "Vagus Nerve as Modulator of the Brain–Gut Axis in Psychiatric and Inflammatory Disorders." 13 March 2018. https://www.frontiersin.org/articles/10.3389/fpsyt.2018.00044/full

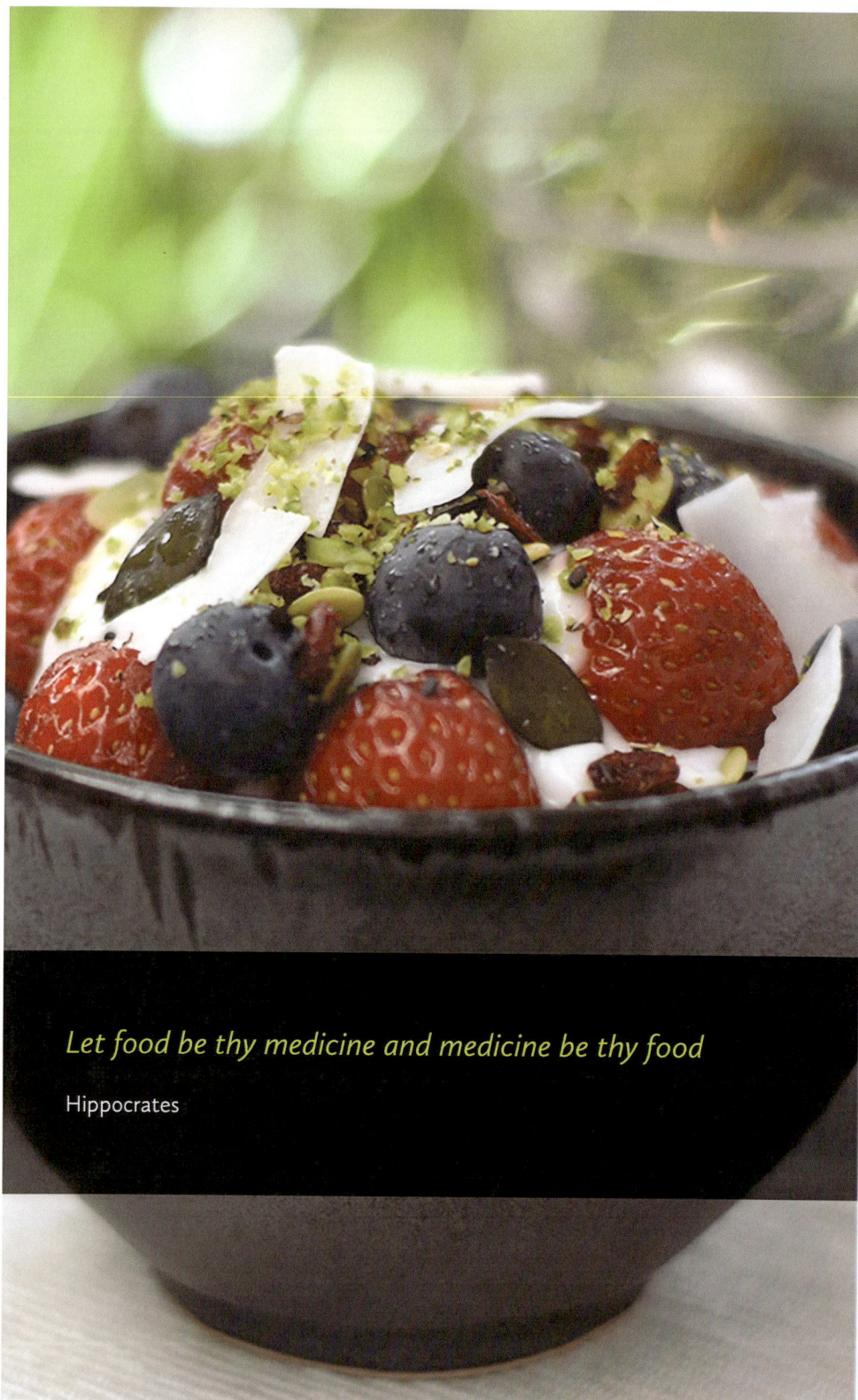

Let food be thy medicine and medicine be thy food

Hippocrates

RESOURCES

Radical Hope
10 Key Healing Factors from Exceptional Survivors of Cancer and other Diseases
Kelly Turner. Hay House 2020

You can also find many more survivor stories on Kelly Turner's Radical Remission website: radicalremission.com

The Cancer-fighting Kitchen
Nourishing, Big-Flavor Recipes for Cancer Treatment and Recovery
Rebecca Katz, Ten Speed Press 2009

The Metabolic Approach to Cancer
Integrating Deep Nutrition, the Ketogenic Diet, and Nontoxic Bio-Individualized Therapies
Dr. Nasha Winters, Jess Higgins Kelley, Kelly Turner (Foreword). Chelsea Green Publishing 2017

The Ketogenic Kitchen
Low carb. High fat. Extraordinary health
Patricia Daly, Nutritional Therapist (dipNT, mBANT, rCNHC), Ocular Melanoma (stage 3c) survivor. Co-written with Domini Kemp, a melanoma and breast cancer survivor). Chelsea Green Publishing 2016

My Answer to Cancer
An Inspirational Story about Life
Cathy Brown. Balboa Press 2016

You Can Conquer Cancer
The ground-breaking self-help manual, including nutrition, meditation and lifestyle management techniques
Ian Gawler. TarcherPerigee 2015

The Ultimate Healthy Home Checklist
Ryan Sternagel

n of 1
One man's Harvard-documented remission of incurable cancer using only natural methods. *Glenn Sabin. Fon Press 2016*

The Golden Path to Natural Healing
Sara Hamo. Createspace 2012

Chris Beat Cancer
A Comprehensive Plan for Healing Naturally
Chris Wark. 2018

Dying to Be Me
My Journey from Cancer, to Near Death, to True Healing
Anita Moorjani. Hay House 2012

The Clever Guts Diet
How to revolutionise your body from the inside out
Dr Michael Mosley. Simon & Schuster 2017

Cancer Survival Strategies
A Holistic Approach
Dr Sandra Cabot. Health Direction 2019

The Longevity Diet
Discover the New Science to slow ageing, fight decease and manage your weight
Dr Valter Longo. Penguin 2018

Vegan Keto
60+ High-Fat Plant Based recipes to nourish your mind & body
Liz MacDowell. Victory Belt Publishing 2018

Feel Better in 5
Your Daily Plan to Feel Great for Life
Dr Rangan Chatterjee. Penguin Life 2019

Phosphorescence: On Awe, Wonder and Things That Sustain You When the World Goes Dark. *Julia Baird. Harper Collins Publishers 2020*

Awe: The New Science of Everyday Wonder and How It Can Transform Your Life," *Dacher Keltner. Penguin Press 2023*

INDEX

Acknowledgements

This book is dedicated to the memory of my beautiful partner and love of my life, who passed away in September 2020 after a long cancer journey.

Her wild spirit now flies free.

I've needed a great deal of support since she passed and while writing this guide. Still do. I knew why I wanted to write it and had the direction fairly clear in my mind but needed plenty of reassurance as it started to take shape. In a way, it has helped me process her loss. I've really appreciated the wonderful support of those who assisted along the way.

I decided to write this book to help others going through a similar journey. We had so many questions going through the cancer journey and it was difficult finding answers. I wish I had known all of the information in this book at the start of that journey but only learned it gradually through a great deal of research and after my partners death.

In particular, I'd like to thank Sue Berry, my partner's Palliative Care Nurse Practitioner. Her patience and support during incredibly challenging times was tender and unwavering.

A sincere thank you to many others who helped on her health journey... Peter Eastman, Trish Banks, Craig Carden, Peter Martin, Wanda Ciu, Jesse Phillips, Ben Thompson as well as all of their support staff - amazing.

Lauren and Ry, my adult daughter and son, a sincere thank you for your deep love and support. I know you're always there for me and without doubt, I'm there for you forever.

My family are so close and supportive of all that I do. I truly am fortunate to have them all, and there's a lot of them! Dad OAM (dec), Mum OAM (dec), Kev, Terry, Michael, (me!), Bernadette, Matt, Ant, Paddy, Phill, Dan, Damien and all of their partners and children. Dan, Pen, (Junee & Flo) live close by and were incredibly supportive throughout it all. Thank you.

Deb Hoadley, a dear friend of my partner, has always been a tremendous support of her (and me!) and has used her extensive writing talents to suggest alterations to my ramblings. Many thanks for your patience.

I promise in future to use fewer exclamation marks!! A big thanks also to those who checked over my writing and provided feedback and suggestions.

A special thank you to all of my partners family and friends who were marvellous in their love and support for both of us. Much love to you all! I also want to thank Diane and Martin Westbrooke, Larissa, Sam and Simon, Belinda and Frank Schaefer, Megan Hallowes, Amanda Collins, Scott Denno, Peter and Michael Nichols, Bun, Barry and Jeannie, Richard Purdy and Jaril.

A huge list of my amazing and supportive friends... To Tim Owen who continually checks in on me and helps me get through - couldn't get by without him, Mr OAM Neville Burrows, a special friend, Rob Soar, another extra special friend and the fella who always knows the right words, and so many more who mean the world to me... Graeme May, Richard & Paula, Dan & Fran, Julie, Jo, Mark, Little, Rosie, Dick, Gem, Aaron, Raylene, Chris's, Joey, Hayles, Ray and Larissa, Lyndal, Jude, Chris and Heather and Emi.

A huge thank you to Diane Foster and Justine Laidlaw who have shown beautiful enthusiasm and appreciation of my bookish efforts. A sincere thank you to you both. You rock!

Thanks also to my devoted and supportive yoga teachers over the years including Tracey, Jill, Bec, Sabrina & Mia - Namaste.

Many others have shown sincere support including Nasha Winter's team, Ted Howard, Chris Wark's team, Glenn Sabin, Ryan Sternagel, Jenny Kennedy, Cathy Brown, Ian Gawler, Sara Hamo and Anita Moorjani's team. Thank you! Nick, Nat & family in beautiful Ocean Grove - thank you!

Everyone at the Community Garden Ocean Grove - awesome!!! Thank you so much for your wonderful support and enthusiasm.

Thank you all! :) xo

About the Author

Paul McKenna is a designer, teacher, university lecturer, photographer and artist and lives in Herne Hill, Victoria, Australia. He has run a design business, Colourfield Design since 2002 working passionately on educational flora and fauna brochures and many other publications and websites. He has worked as an Experience Designer, lectured in Design Skills, User Experience Design and Design Thinking at Deakin University and has worked in the Web Team at Federation University.

He has two adult children he's very proud of and loves dearly. You can often find him at home in the lush garden tending the veggies and native plants and smelling the roses. Oh, and he likes the beach.

He is ever grateful for his large, boisterous, crazy and wonderful family of nine brothers and one sister and most importantly an amazing Mum OAM (dec) who taught him to 'never give up' and 'look after others'. His Dad OAM (dec) spent his life looking after his family and making the world a better place. Two wonderful role models.

He is constantly inspired by the hard work and dedication of the many in the medical field who tirelessly support cancer patients and those passionate about holistic and natural approaches.

He hopes people will find hope, peace, reassurance and empowerment reading this book in their time of need.

Contact

I welcome your feedback on the book.

Ideally, I want the guide to be the best possible support for those newly diagnosed with cancer or on the cancer journey. You're welcome to contact me using the following details.

empowering.au
Email: paul@empowering.au

I wish you all the best
Paul McKenna

www.ingramcontent.com/pod-product-compliance
Lightning Source LLC
Chambersburg PA
CBRC101141030426
42334CB00012B/125